Contents

3

Preface

Over 270,000 new patients are diagnosed with cancer annually in the UK which represents an increase of approximately 2.8% for men and 4.4% for women between 1991 and 2000.[1] Over the same period significant improvements in survival have been achieved and indeed there has been a 12% reduction in cancer mortality within the last decade.[2] As a result there has been a considerable increase in the number of patients living with cancer, currently estimated to be around 1.2 million in the U.K.[1]

It is now clearly established that imaging is central to the management of patients with cancer throughout the patient pathway and it is not surprising therefore that there has been a relentless increase in the demand for oncological imaging during recent years. Much has been achieved through the implementation of the *NHS Cancer Plan* [3,4] with major investment in imaging equipment over the last decade, but increased pressure on radiology departments for general as well as for cancer imaging has resulted in longer waiting times for cross-sectional imaging. The introduction of cancer targets *[maximum two month (62 days) wait from urgent GP referral to first treatment for all cancers by December 2005; maximum one month (31 days) wait from decision to treat to first definitive treatment for all cancers by December 2005][2,5]* has highlighted the importance of improving access to imaging for cancer patients and has thereby stimulated the need to introduce up-to-date national cancer imaging guidance.

This document has been produced to provide guidelines and protocols for computed tomography (CT) and magnetic resonance imaging (MRI) in cancer with the objective of helping to achieve a high quality, efficient and uniform cancer imaging service across the UK. A major advantage of adopting national protocols is the ability to provide a streamlined effective service in which appropriate scans are undertaken according to the patient's tumour type and purpose of the examination. These protocols will also ensure that imaging studies can be compared more accurately during follow-up in an individual patient, irrespective of where the patient has been imaged. This is particularly important for reducing the need to repeat imaging of patients being entered into clinical trials.

CT and MRI are used at all stages of the patient pathway: diagnosis, staging, determining the appropriate therapy, including eligibility to enter into clinical trials, and during follow-up. Cross-sectional imaging is also used for the assessment of residual disease and for determining the presence and extent of tumour relapse. These key roles were recognised by previous editions of this manual,[6,7] but guidelines and protocols need to be continually appraised and updated to keep abreast of technological advances and new therapeutic approaches so that optimum results can be achieved. This document complements the recent publication *Imaging for Oncology* published by the Royal College of Radiologists in 2004.[8] The current edition brings CT and MRI together within the same document, reflecting the current clinical practice of these complementary techniques. We have included reference to the role of [18]FDG PET-CT for staging and assessment of malignancy and have also indicated those situations in which [18]FDG PET does not appear to be useful at the present time. These guidelines are intended to provide practical advice and recommendations which should be achievable for the majority of patients. However, they are not intended to be prescriptive and could be adapted readily to meet local requirements.

4

We have not included information on image interpretation which can be found in many excellent textbooks, journals and internet resources. We have tried to follow as closely as possible a standardised page layout, including reference to the TNM classification of tumours, where appropriate. The guidelines have been written with a view to future developments in clinical practice and therefore indications for ^{18}F 2-Fluorodeoxyglucose positron emission tomography with CT anatomical fusion (^{18}FDG PET-CT) and Hydrogen MR spectroscopy (MRS) are included. We have assumed that the majority of radiology departments have access to multislice CT (MSCT) and to MRI equipment operating at 1.5 tesla for imaging cancer patients; for the few departments that do not currently have access to these technologies, protocols will need to be adapted accordingly.

The Royal College of Radiologists has brought together a panel of nationally and internationally recognised radiologists with particular expertise in cancer imaging to produce these recommendations. All the contributors work in busy radiology departments within the NHS with a large cancer patient referral base. I would like to thank all those who have contributed to the document for their hard work and dedication and, in particular, I would like to express my gratitude to Dr. Anwar Padhani who has taken a leading role in bringing this project to fruition. I would also like to thank Mrs Maureen Watts for her expert administrative support for this project.

We hope that these protocols will be used widely within departments of radiology undertaking cancer imaging and will help to improve cancer services across the UK.

Janet Husband

Janet E. Husband, OBE FMedSci FRCP PRCR
Chairman of Working Party
President, Royal College of Radiologists

References:

1.   Tom JR (ed). *CancerStats Monograph 2004*. Cancer Research UK, London, 2004. ISBN: 0-9546256-2-5

2.   *The NHS cancer plan and the new NHS: Providing a patient-centred service.* Dept. of Health, 27/10/2004; www.dh.gov.uk/publications

3.   *The NHS Cancer plan: a plan for investment, a plan for reform.* Dept. of Health, 27/9/2000; www.dh.gov.uk/publications

4.   *The NHS Cancer Plan: Making progress.* Dept. of Health, 03/12/2001; www.dh.gov.uk/publications

5.   *Cancer waiting targets: A guide (Version 4).* Dept. of Health, 22/7/05; www.dh.gov.uk/publications

6.   *The Use of Computed Tomography in the Initial Investigation of Common Malignancies.* The Royal College of Radiologists, London, 1995; RCR Ref. No. RCR(95)1.

7.   *A Guide to the Practical Use of MRI in Oncology.* The Royal College of Radiologists, London, 1999; RCR Ref. No. BFCR(99)6

8.   *Imaging for Oncology: Collaboration between clinical radiologists and clinical oncologists in diagnosis, staging and radiotherapy planning.* The Royal College of Radiologists, London, 2004; RCR Ref. No. BFCO(04)2

CHAPTER 1

Imaging in the evaluation of cancer

Introduction

Cross-sectional imaging has a central role to play in the management of patients with malignant disease and is used at all points along the patient pathway:

a) In the initial diagnosis and the staging of disease extent.

b) For monitoring response to treatment.

c) For evaluation of any residual mass after treatment.

d) For confirmation of remission of disease.

e) For recognition of complications of treatment.

f) When there is concern for disease relapse.

CT and MR imaging have well recognised strengths and weaknesses. At different points along the patient pathway one or other may be more appropriately used depending upon whether treatment intent is curative or palliative, and whether the imaging focus is for local or metastatic disease. There are a number of practical steps which ensure good practice in cancer imaging:

- The provision in the request form of all clinical information relating to histological diagnosis, site of disease, previous surgery or other treatment and the specific purpose of the examination. All CT and MR requests in patients with known or suspected cancer should be vetted by radiologists or experienced radiographers.

- There are considerations about the timing of staging investigation after surgery. After dissection of the neck, groin or axilla, there may be a complex residual mass. After resection of a bladder tumour there may be reactive changes which mimic tumour spread. It is vital that the radiologist is fully appraised of the date and nature of surgery performed prior to staging. Where possible, a delay after surgery will allow these changes to resolve.

- All previous radiological investigations should be available or be retrievable in an electronic form for review by the radiologist responsible prior to the examination.

- Although routine patients should be scanned according to standard protocols, examinations may need to be tailored to answer specific questions. Each department should have written, well-defined protocols for standard examinations.

- Where possible, examinations should be reviewed before the patient leaves the department to ensure that the examination is technically satisfactory and to assess the need for additional imaging. Review is aided by preset centre / window functions on the diagnostic console for soft tissue, liver, lung, brain and bone. The final report should be issued only after interrogation of the images on all relevant settings on the diagnostic console.

- Radiologists should be familiar with the normal range of appearances on their equipment as this varies considerably on different machines.

- Lymph nodes should be measured in the short axis in the axial plane. Normal lymph node sizes (maximum short axis dimensions – MSAD) for different anatomical areas are presented in chapter 3.

- Since response to treatment and disease progression are assessed according to changes in tumour size, follow-up examinations should be performed with comparable technique using the same planes and sequences. Ideally, both sets of examinations should be available to the radiologists 'side by side' on the diagnostic console.

- Although there is a great variation in style of reporting, it is good practice to provide a succinct conclusion, paying attention to answering the specific clinical question posed. (See the section below in this chapter on reporting.) Recommendations regarding follow-up, biopsy and alternative radiological studies should also be made in the conclusion.

- It should be possible to review all relevant examinations in a multidisciplinary meeting, especially when there is discrepancy between clinical and imaging findings or other diagnostic uncertainty.

Principles of cancer staging

A clinically useful classification scheme for cancer encompasses the attributes of the cancer and defines its behaviour. Current schemes are based on the premise that cancers of the same histological type arising in the same anatomical location share similarities in patterns of growth and spread, and have similar outcomes. The process of staging determines how widely a cancer has spread. Clinical staging is performed in patients when there is a reasonable likelihood that a cancer has metastasised. Staging information is used in several ways:

a) For selection of the primary and adjuvant therapies.

b) For estimating patient prognosis.

c) To assist in the evaluation of the success of therapy.

d) To facilitate the exchange of information between providers of healthcare and between treatment centres.

e) To contribute to the knowledge base of investigations into the behaviour and treatment of cancer.

Key points in cancer staging

- Although clinical examinations, blood tests and simple imaging such as chest radiographs and ultrasound can reveal much useful information, detailed cross-sectional imaging and scintigraphy are the key elements of the staging process. 18^{FDG} PET-CT is an important, evolving technology for staging selected tumours.

- In most patients staging follows histological diagnosis of the primary tumour, and in some situations there are histological analyses of regional lymph node status and distant sites. In other patients imaging diagnosis precedes histological confirmation and it may replace histological confirmation of the extent of disease spread.

- It should be noted that staging is different for tumours with different histology in the same organ, e.g., renal cell cancer and transitional cell cancer of the kidney. Different information is required to plan the different treatment options for the two tumours and the different patterns of metastasis.

- Staging is a process of detection and exclusion. Only those regions of the body which are commonly and predictably involved by the individual tumour should be examined.

- Staging requires the use of the best possible imaging modalities available and should be performed in the fewest steps. This minimises inconvenience for patients and the delay between diagnosis and the beginning of treatment.

- If patients are unfit for radical therapy, only information required to guide palliative therapy should be obtained.

- Staging should be performed according to agreed protocols, but procedures must be flexible to accommodate unusual presentations of disease and individual patient needs (e.g., patients who are physically or mentally challenged).

- The choice of imaging modalities used may require compromise. Factors to be considered include: local availability and expertise, tolerance of the staging investigations by the patient and patient convenience.

- A single test is preferred to multiple investigations. The ability to rapidly and reproducibly examine large tissue volumes makes CT the preferred option for staging patients with metastatic disease.

- It should be understood that exclusion of metastasis is never absolute; it is important that all those involved in patient management recognise the limitations of imaging investigations.

Limitations of staging

Lesion threshold

For every test there is a threshold above which disease is considered present and below which it is considered absent. This threshold represents a compromise. For example, a threshold for lymph nodes frequently used is 10 mm for maximum short axis dimension (MSAD). Nevertheless, nodes greater than this are frequently benign and nodes smaller than 10 mm may contain metastases.

The thresholds used may vary according to the implications for treatment (e.g., to optimise diagnostic accuracy or according to treatment intent). Thus, using a treatment protocol that requires removal of nodes that are **definitely** considered metastatic, a higher threshold is appropriate (thereby improving specificity by reducing the number of reactive nodes removed) than if using a treatment protocol that requires aggressive removal of all **potentially** metastatic (which would improve sensitivity – but at the cost of reduced specificity).

Detection and characterisation

There is a difference between detection and characterisation of a lesion. Although chest radiography will reveal most lung nodules of more than 10 mm in diameter, some may be missed in "hidden" lung regions, e.g., the lung apex or behind the heart. The technical and diagnostic advantages of CT are its ability to reveal small nodules down to the size of approximately 3 mm and nodules which are invisible on chest radiography. However, it should be noted that there are also "hidden" areas on CT (particularly in the perihilar regions) which are frequently missed, and that small lesions (less than 1 cm) are usually too small to characterise. Indeterminate small lesions are also frequent in other anatomical sites within the body, for example, the liver.

Indeterminate lesions; management of uncertainty

Indeterminate lesions should be the subject of clinico-radiological discussion and/or multidisciplinary review, if establishment of their nature would impact upon patient management. If an indeterminate lesion was present on comparable imaging studies prior to the diagnosis, then stability over more than 6 months usually indicates it is benign. If there is another diagnostic test which is likely to provide a definitive diagnosis, this should be performed. Biopsy is rarely an option for lesions less than 10 mm in size. Sometimes, the only practical option available is "watchful waiting", to monitor the behaviour of the lesion over time. A wait and watch policy without treatment is appropriate when a patient is asymptomatic or when active management would not be prejudiced by a delay in lesion characterisation.

Thus the options for resolving uncertainties about staging include:

a) Discussion.
b) Further investigation.
c) Intervention.
d) Active monitoring (wait and watch).

Multidisciplinary team meetings

Multidisciplinary team (MDT) meetings permit a team approach to patient management in which all aspects of the patient's disease are considered in order to provide optimum therapy. Selection of cases for inclusion and evaluation of responses within clinical trials and provision of a framework for continuing professional development, audit and multidisciplinary research are also key objectives.

For most patients the information provided by staging confirms the clinical impression of disease extent. However, in a minority of patients there are discrepancies between the clinical impression and imaging findings or other problems requiring further discussion. Clinicians and radiologists need to identify problem cases which should be reviewed in advance. Following MDT meetings, the results of reviews, including discrepancies with previous findings, must be documented in clinical notes and, if necessary, in addendum to radiology reports. Any further investigations required should be instigated promptly. Feedback should be available to all radiologists within referring Cancer Units. The time required by radiologists to undertake all these activities should be recognised in job planning. MDT meetings should be supported by appropriate clerical and administrative staff, and all individuals necessary to sanction investigations and to execute treatment plans should attend. Facilities should be available for televisual projection and display of relevant pathology and radiology, as determined by local needs.

Staging systems

A variety of staging systems are used in clinical practice. Staging schemes are based on the premise that cancers arising from the same anatomical locations and sharing similar histological features will have similarities in their patterns of growth and ultimate outcomes. Staging systems define tumour extent which, in turn, determines treatment options and provides a guide to prognosis.

The most widely used system is the TNM system of UICC[1] (International Union Against Cancer) and this scheme has been wholly adopted by the American Joint Committee on Cancer (AJCC).[2] However, other systems have been defined by professional organisations and institutions for specific tumours or groups of tumours for which the TNM staging system does not exist or is inappropriate (e.g., paediatric, brain, lymphoma, pleural mesothelioma, testicular and ovarian). For local radiological practice, it is important that the staging systems used are well understood and uniformly applied by all in a clinical team.

In the TNM system an alphanumeric annotation defines the following:

T Stage The local disease extent with the use of numerical subsets which indicates the progressive extent of the malignant process (T0, T1, T2, T3, T4).

N Stage Nodal status which indicates the presence or absence of regional lymph node metastasis(es) (N0, N1, N2, N3)

M Stage Metastasis stage which defines the presence or absence of distant metastasis (M0, M1)

Description of the general rules for the TNM classification and the documentation of specific classification for individual tumours are beyond the scope of this document. All readers are strongly encouraged to have at the bench side either the *TNM Atlas* of the UICC or the *Cancer Staging Handbook* of the AJCC, where the appropriate guidance and definitions can be found readily.[1,2]

Reporting

The imaging report should comprise the following components:

Indication: a statement regarding clinical or surgical staging, pathology and tumour marker levels, if relevant and available.

Technique: details of contrast medium administered and imaging parameters used (including sequences) to allow exact replication on follow-up examinations.

Findings: a concise statement on imaging findings, including clear identification of marker lesions by anatomic location, size (by measurement) and imaging section(s) (by slice number(s) or table position). The presence of complications such as bowel obstruction, hydronephrosis or venous thrombosis should be stated.

When a comparison has been made with a previous examination, the date of examination (and place, if from another institution) should be indicated.

Impression or conclusion: if possible, this should provide a staging assessment (TNM status or other) highlighting categories of uncertainty, where appropriate, by the use of the relevant TNM prefix TX, NX, MX. Recommendations regarding follow-up, biopsy and alternative radiological studies should also be made in the conclusion.

Imaging the treated patient

Reproducibility is a key factor in providing accurate assessment of response. Thus, follow-up imaging techniques and protocols should be identical to those used for the initial staging, provided that the initial examination was optimal.

Investigation of suspected relapse should be tailored to the clinical presentation and the anticipated treatment intent. Patients may relapse outside compartments or areas of the body treated initially with surgery or radiotherapy and, therefore, follow-up study protocols may need to be adapted to examine different areas from the initial staging examination. When relapse is suspected, a patient's ability to tolerate the examination may be compromised by symptoms, and it may be helpful to discuss the proposed examination with the clinical team prior to the study. Patients, for instance, with bowel obstruction may not tolerate oral contrast media.

Documentation of response to treatment

Imaging reports of patients undergoing treatment should document changes in tumour size, using criteria agreed between the radiologist and oncologist and/or as required by clinical trial protocols.

For many years the WHO response criteria devised in 1981[3] were used for assessment of treatment response. These criteria are well understood and simple to apply by radiologists and clinicians alike. They are entirely reasonable to use in clinical practice, particularly in patients not entered into clinical trials.

More recently the RECIST *(Response Criteria in Solid Tumours)* criteria have been devised.[4] The RECIST criteria are designed to be used in clinical trials and require measurement and documentation of multiple sites of cancer. This work is highly demanding of radiologists' time and, since it represents clinical research, cannot be considered to constitute routine work.

WHO criteria - Definitions of objective response[3]	
Complete response (CR)	Disappearance of all known disease
Partial response (PR)	50% or more decrease in total tumour load (single or multiple lesions, bidimensional or unidimensional measurement)
No change (NC)	50% decrease or 25% increase not established
Progressive disease (PD)	25% or more increase in the size of measurable lesion or appearance of new lesions

Note: Bidimensional measurements are used resulting in an area product

Using the RECIST criteria the disease burden is classified into measurable and non-measurable lesions. Measurable disease is classified into target and non-target lesions. Lesions are required to be >1 cm in single long axis dimension on CT. No more than 5 target lesions per organ are chosen, and full assessment requires a maximum of 10 target lesions per patient. All lesions require reassessment at each attendance. The final response assessment category requires an assessment of both measurable and non-measurable disease. The lesion sum length is used in the response assessment. Non-measurable lesions include all lesions less than 1 cm in single long axis dimension, ascites, bone lesions, pleural / pericardial effusions, etc.[4]

RECIST criteria[4]	
Complete response (CR)	Disappearance of all target lesions, confirmed at 4 weeks
Partial response (PR)	At least a 30% decrease in the sum of the longest diameter of target lesions, taking as reference the baseline sum of the longest diameter, confirmed at 4 weeks
No change (NC)	Neither sufficient shrinkage to qualify for partial response nor sufficient increase to qualify for progressive disease
Progressive disease (PD)	At least a 20% increase in the sum of the longest diameter of target lesions, taking as reference the smallest sum of the longest diameter recorded since the treatment started or the appearance of one or more new lesions

There are a number of concerns about the RECIST criteria which are relevant to reporting of imaging studies:[5]

a) The use of the axial plane is required by RECIST. However, lesions can often be better defined in other planes using MRI and multi-planar reconstructions of CT data. Lymph node enlargement may be mainly in the longitudinal plane, particularly in confined regions such as the retroperitoneum.

b) Long axis measurements can be problematic; e.g., en plaque tumour growth (short axis measurements may be more reproducible).

c) Lymph node dimensions in CT and MR are recommended in the short axis (MSAD), and the use of longest dimensions leads to additional work and may lead to confusion, particularly for those entering data into case report forms.

d) Cystic tumours are excluded (i.e., non-measurable disease) yet cystic changes can be key indicators of response and define management for conditions such as germ cell tumours.

e) Bone metastases, some of which can be accurately defined and measured with MR imaging, are excluded.

f) It is not clear what to do about lesions that are initially measurable and subsequently become non-measurable with treatment; this can happen in the context of both disease response and progression.

g) There is no conformity in windowing of lesions for measurement when, in fact, lesions may differ in size at different window settings.

h) Use of the lesion sum length may disguise differential responses.

i) The number of scans prescribed, their frequency and the rigid prescription of body parts to be examined may be at variance with good practice, particularly in respect of ionizing radiation dose (e.g., for children and young adults with curable cancers).

j) There are significant concerns about the increase in workload.

A number of theoretical and non-radiological concerns also exist. The need to measure 10 lesions is without a firm evidence base and, indeed, one study has shown that measurement of more than two lesions does not add value to the clinical trials process.[6] The threshold of 20% linear increase in lesion size before diagnosis of progressive disease will artificially increase the number of patients with stable disease (the actual equivalent figure would be a 12% increase, if parity is to be maintained with the older WHO criteria of 30%). For these and other considerations, comparison of data between trials using WHO and RECIST assessments is problematic, but most trials now use RECIST.

However, notwithstanding the limitations outlined above, the vast majority of current clinical trials use RECIST as the standard. A practical approach is summarised below:

- Unidimensional assessment.
- Measurement of up to ten lesions to determine response (in practice, four is a reasonable compromise).
- Note that no measurements are necessary if a new metastatic lesion is seen, as this is unequivocal disease progression.

Imaging plays a major role in the follow-up of residual masses. A residual mass is generally defined as a post-treatment mass greater than 1 cm in diameter, but in non-Hodgkin's lymphoma and Hodgkin's lymphoma a residual mass is classified as a nodal mass 1.5 cm in diameter or greater.[7] The imaging strategies used will vary with different tumour types. Residual lymphoma masses are typically subject to repeated imaging, while non-seminomatous germ cell tumour residual masses are frequently resected. An evolving imaging technique to confirm stability is [18]FDG PET-CT which has been shown to be reliable for distinguishing active from inactive disease within the residual mass in many tumour types.[8,9]

References:

1.   Sobin LH, Whittekind CH (Eds). *TNM Classification of Malignant Tumours*.
        6th ed. New York: Wiley-Liss; 2002.

2.   Greene FL, Page DL, Fleming ID, et al., (Eds). *AJCC Cancer Staging Handbook*.
        TNM classification of malignant tumours. 6th ed. New York: Springer-Verlag, 2002.

3.   Miller AB, Hoogstraten B, Staquet M, Winkler A. Reporting results of cancer treatment.
        Cancer 1981; 47: 207-14.

4.   Therasse P, Arbuck SG, Eisenhauer EA, et al. New guidelines to evaluate the response to treatment
        in solid tumours. European Organization for Research and Treatment of Cancer, National Cancer
        Institute of United States, National Cancer Institute of Canada. *J Natl Cancer* Inst 2000; 92: 205-216.

5.   Husband JE, Schwartz LH, Spencer J, et al. Evaluation of the response to treatment of solid tumours
        – a consensus statement of the International Cancer Imaging Society. *Br J Cancer* 2004; 90: 2256-2260.

6.   Hillman SL, Sargent DJ, An M-W, et al. Evaluation of RECIST criteria in determining the response to
        treatment in solid tumors: A North Central Cancer Treatment Group (NCCTG) investigation.
        Proc Am Soc Clin Oncol 2003; 22, p 521 (abstract 2095).

7.   Cheson BD, Horning SJ, Coiffier B, et al. Report of an international workshop to standardize
        response criteria for non-Hodgkin's lymphomas. NCI Sponsored   International Working Group.
        J Clin Oncol 1999; 17: 1244.

8.   Lavely WC, Delbeke D, Greer JP, et al. FDG PET in the follow-up management of patients with newly
        diagnosed Hodgkin and non-Hodgkin lymphoma after first-line chemotherapy.
        Int J Radiat Oncol Biol Phys 2003; 57: 307-315.

9.   Hain SF, O'Doherty MJ, Timothy AR, et al. Fluorodeoxyglucose positron emission tomography in the
        evaluation of germ cell tumours at relapse. *Br J Cancer* 2000; 83: 863-869.

CHAPTER 2

General techniques for examinations

Computed Tomography (CT)

Patient preparation

It is helpful for patients to receive general information about the scan prior to attendance in the department, and this is best achieved in leaflet or booklet form. The information should include a brief description of CT scanning, the specific preparation that will be required, the time taken for the examination, including waiting time in the department, and a statement about to whom and when the report will be sent. The use of intravenous contrast medium for the majority of CT examinations should also be included.

At the time of attendance it is useful to check that out-patients have an appropriate clinic appointment.

For abdomino-pelvic examinations it is usual to ask the patient to fast for 4 hours.

It is important to be aware of patients with renal impairment and to take measures to minimise contrast medium nephrotoxicity (CMN). Patients at risk should receive a small dose of either non-ionic iso-osmolar dimeric or non-ionic low osmolar monomeric contrast medium and intravenous fluid. Intravenous infusion (1 ml/kg patient body weight/h) of 0.9% saline starting 4 hours before contrast injection and continuing for at least 12 hours afterwards is effective in reducing the incidence of CMN.[1]

Patient positioning

Patients are usually scanned supine with their arms raised above the head for CT of the torso. Any variations are detailed in the text.

Contrast medium

Bowel opacification

- Bowel contrast medium is generally given in the form of a water-soluble iodine or a diluted barium-based agent. For general abdomino-pelvic CT examinations, one litre of dilute oral contrast medium is recommended. This is given in divided doses commencing 1 hour before the scan with the last dose of approximately 150-200 ml being given immediately before the patient is positioned on the scanner. A smaller volume of contrast medium is required for limited upper abdominal studies (approximately 500 ml).

- Contrast opacification of the colon and rectum can be improved by administration of a small dose of oral contrast medium 4-12 hours before the examination. For out-patients, this can be achieved by sending a small vial of contrast through the post with the appointment letter and information leaflet. 5 ml of Gastrografin taken in 150-200 ml of water is effective, if taken last thing at night for morning examinations or after breakfast for afternoon appointments.

- Some in-patients receive their oral contrast on the ward. Effective administration is encouraged by liaison between skilled radiographic helpers and ward staff. Some patients prefer flavourings in the contrast medium. The radiologist / radiographer should ensure that these flavourings do not result in precipitation of the contrast medium within the bowel lumen.

- Rectal contrast medium is not mandatory but may assist in the delineation of disease within the pelvis. If used, 100 ml is suggested followed by 50 ml of air which helps to push the contrast medium into the sigmoid colon.

- Water and carbon dioxide granules may also be used as oral contrast agents (particularly for staging examinations of the stomach and oesophagus - see chapters 8 and 11).

- If bowel opacification is suboptimal, then delayed scans, with or without additional oral contrast medium, or scans with the patient in the decubitus or prone position, may be useful.

- Prior to abdominal CT, it is important to check that the patient has not had a recent barium study since retained, radiographically dense barium will degrade the images by streak artefacts.

Intravenous contrast medium

- The use of intravenous contrast medium (IVCM) is an important component of the CT examination. Each intravenous injection should be planned to maximise positive information from the scan and minimise risk and discomfort to the patient.

- The information to be derived from the CT examination should determine the intravenous technique to be used. Contrast medium should be given as a rapid intravenous bolus via an intravenous (IV) cannula using a pump injector. It is advisable that CT departments adhere to established protocols, and radiographic staff should make themselves familiar with them. With appropriate training and supervision, placement of the IV cannula, injection of contrast and aftercare management of the cannula site can all be delegated to radiographic and/or nursing staff.

- Spiral CT allows examination of large volumes of the body within a single breathhold. With single slice spiral CT for general examination of the abdomen and pelvis in a single breathhold, the technique requires approximately 100-150 ml of 300 mg iodine strength contrast medium, administered at 3-4 ml/sec, beginning the examination in the portal venous phase of enhancement at 65-70 seconds after commencement of the injection. When the chest is examined a first breathhold acquisition at 25-30 seconds after commencement of injection is followed by the abdomino-pelvic acquisition in a second breathhold. For general examinations of the torso, slice thicknesses of 5-10 mm are used with single slice CT. Details of slice thicknesses and contrast protocols which differ from these general statements are indicated in the relevant chapters.

- With multislice (multidetector) CT (MSCT or MDCT) the options for imaging parameters are even wider than single slice. The same principles apply for timing of CT acquisitions relative to injection of IVCM, although the short acquisition times mean that there is a greater chance of the acquisition 'missing' the contrast bolus due to variations in cardiac output between patients. Bolus tracking techniques can minimise this risk.

- For examination of the brain 50-100 ml of 300 mg iodine strength contrast medium should be administered; the rate of injection and the timing of the scan in relation to the injection are less critical than for body CT.

Imaging parameters for spiral CT

- Using MDCT there is a trade-off between volume and speed of coverage and contrast and spatial resolution in terms of collimation and dose of ionising radiation. For example, in breathless or restless individuals large volumes of coverage can be achieved which would previously have been impossible or exquisite anatomical detail of a region of interest can be obtained.

- MDCT allows near isotropic imaging and with selection of appropriate imaging parameters, high quality multiplanar reconstructions (MPR) and 3-D renderings are possible. Data can be reconstructed at different slice thicknesses from 1-10 mm. Overlapping reconstructions of data further improve image quality and for most available machines 2-3 mm overlapping reconstructions of the abdomen and pelvis result in high quality renderings.

- CT cancer staging should not be performed on conventional, incremental CT scanners.

Radiation protection for the patient in CT

Notwithstanding the undoubted role of properly directed CT scanning in the clinical management of cancer patients, the levels of potentially harmful radiation delivered to the patient can be relatively high when compared to many other types of diagnostic x-ray examination.[2] There is consequently a need to balance the benefits and risks from CT within the broad context of a patient's health, both present and future, through active management of patient dose.[3] In principle, this means the elimination of all unnecessary radiation exposure. In practice, it requires the prior clinical justification of all CT examinations and the use of optimal scanning techniques that result in the lowest patient dose to meet each particular clinical purpose. These guiding principles for radiation protection are enshrined in European and UK legislation.[4,5]

Once duly authorised by the practitioner or operator,[5] each CT examination should be conducted by the application of protocols developed for specific clinical purposes by the radiographer and radiologist (in close collaboration with the medical physics expert when needed). Such protocols should reflect good scanning practice, with active management of technique including:

- tube current,
- x-ray beam collimation,
- pitch,
- length of each scan sequence, and
- number of such sequences.

Attention to these factors will limit the patient dose to the minimum level commensurate with providing the diagnostic information required. Significant reductions in dose can be achieved, for example, by utilising the technology available with newer scanner models for the automatic modulation of tube current according to patient anatomy.[6] Many scanner models also display values of the two practical dose quantities, volume CT dose index ($CTDI_{vol}$) and dose-length product (DLP), which have been defined for the purpose of promoting the use of good technique. Levels of such doses should be assessed for each protocol and, as an initial step in the process of optimisation, compared against relevant national reference doses that are published by the Radiation Protection Division of the Health Protection Agency (formerly the National Radiological Protection Board), following periodic reviews of national practice.[7] The 2003 national reference values for $CTDI_{vol}$ are summarised for various scan regions and patient groups in the Appendix. These doses are intended to represent levels to trigger the investigation of potentially unacceptable practice. Consequently, any local levels of dose above the relevant national reference dose should be reviewed for potential changes in technique that could lead to dose reduction without compromising clinical requirements.

Since children are potentially more susceptible to radiation effects, special attention should be given to the justification and optimisation of paediatric CT scanning. Particular regard should be given to the use of size-specific scan protocols and dose reduction software, where this is available.

Biopsy

If CT is the preferred technique for guiding the biopsy, good practice dictates that prior to beginning the biopsy procedure:

a) informed consent is obtained,

b) the possibility of a bleeding diathesis is excluded or corrected,

c) provision is made for aftercare, e.g., a day care bed,

d) there is liaison with colleagues in the histopathology/cytology departments so that preservation and storage of tissue are appropriate or a member of the cytology department is present at the procedure to assess the adequacy of the material obtained from a fine needle aspiration, and

e) a diagnostic CT scan is undertaken with intravenous contrast medium to assess both the vascularity of the lesion and its relationship to adjacent vessels. This scan is also useful for planning the patient position, determining lesion choice and biopsy route.

Where possible, needle core biopsy should be obtained. Use of 18G needles is usually sufficient.

It should be remembered that sampling errors, although small, are not insignificant. If the clinical features are overwhelmingly those of malignancy, but this is not supported by the histopathology, then the biopsy should be repeated, perhaps from a different anatomical location or the patient referred for surgical biopsy. Only a biopsy result positive for cancer is reliable in the short-term; negative biopsies only being corroborated by follow-up.

Radiation protection for patients and staff during CT biopsy procedures

Needle guidance during biopsy may be undertaken using conventional CT imaging or CT fluoroscopy (CTF). The latter technology provides real-time images, although there is potential for significantly higher doses to the patient from continuous localised exposure and to staff (particularly in relation to eyes, thyroid and hands) from their close proximity to the x-ray beam during needle manipulation.[8]

There is a particular need for active dose management during CTF in order to limit screening times and tube currents to the minimum values necessary and, when manipulating the needle during real-time imaging, to keep hands away from the x-ray beam. The use of special needle holders and lead sheets placed over the patient can help reduce hand exposures. Doses to both patients and staff are also reduced when CTF is used intermittently as a series of very short exposures in a 'quick-check' mode between needle manipulations, rather than in 'real-time' mode with simultaneous needle manipulation and CTF.[9]

Magnetic Resonance Imaging (MRI)

Patient preparation

All patients should be sent an information leaflet or booklet at the time of booking their appointment. The booklet should include a brief description of the MRI scanner and of the need to place coils closer to the body to improve the pictures obtained. Patients should be made aware of the loud noise which occurs during scanning and earplugs should be available. The use of intramuscular and intravenous injections should be mentioned as well as the expected overall duration of the examination. Booklets should also include a list of absolute contraindications to MRI in a language style appropriate to patients. Patients should be provided with a telephone number to discuss possible concerns about safety aspects. When there are concerns for intra-ocular or other relevant metallic fragments, the patient may need to attend in advance of the MRI appointment for radiographs / limited CT scans.

Concerns about claustrophobia can be addressed by encouraging the patient to visit the MRI unit before the study is undertaken so that fears relating to the examination can be allayed as far as possible. Approximately 1-2% of patients are unable to proceed due to claustrophobia and some patients may require sedation. Sedation should always be given in accordance with Royal College of Radiologists' guidelines,[10] and be organised in advance of the appointment to enable the procedure to be conducted in a relaxed and orderly manner. Sedation can be by oral pre-medication or by intravenous injection. There must be appropriate monitoring equipment and aftercare for sedated patients, and national guidelines as well as local rules must be followed in this regard.

On arrival in the department the scanning procedures should be explained to the patient by a specialist radiographer. This should include a discussion on the use of various coils and whether an intravenous injection will be required for the study.

The patient should be asked about any contraindications to MRI and about the possibility of pregnancy; a checklist is recommended which the patient is then asked to sign.

Patient handling

Patients are usually scanned in the supine position, but in those patients who are claustrophobic, the prone position has been found to be helpful. The patient's arms are usually placed by their side and quiet respiration is permitted for all examinations except those where breathhold techniques are used. An intramuscular or intravenous bowel relaxant (Hyoscine-N-Butyl Bromide (Buscopan) or Glucagon) may be required for some abdominal / pelvic MRI examinations to reduce bowel peristalsis.

Sequences

Although there are a large number of different sequences used for MRI examinations and different manufacturers use different terminology for the same sequences, discussion of all these different approaches is considered inappropriate in this document. In general, T1-weighted (T1W) and fast/turbo spin-echo T2-weighted (T2W) sequences are used for the evaluation of tumours. Fat suppression either using a frequency selective saturation pulse or short tau inversion recovery (STIR) is also valuable. Gradient-echo sequences may be employed for in- and opposed-phase imaging and to obtain rapid data acquisition, particularly when using three-dimensional (3-D) and breath-hold contrast-enhanced techniques.

Respiratory compensation, navigator assistance and pre-saturation pulses for abdominal imaging are all helpful when used appropriately. Cardiac gating is also valuable for both chest and abdominal studies to reduce pulsatile motion artefact.

Supervision of oncological MRI examinations by a trained MR radiologist or radiographer is vital to ensure that adequate image quality and satisfactory diagnostic information are obtained.

Field of view / matrix

The field of view and matrix size are inter-related, as the matrix size used varies according to the field of view used. The aim is to produce high resolution images with adequate signal-to-noise ratio of the organ or area of interest, and these parameters will depend upon the equipment used as well as other factors such as the size of the primary tumour or organ being studied. High resolution, small field of view T2W images in two planes are required for most pelvic examinations. Some organs such as the prostate gland have predictable orientation; others such as the uterus and cervix show a greater variation in anatomical position and therefore require prescription of oblique planes to ensure maximal diagnostic information.

Coils

While the body coil is suitable for imaging large areas of the body, e.g., for survey of the whole abdomen or pelvis or for localisation of organs prior to detailed examination, local tumour staging should be undertaken using surface or endocavitary coils.

A wide range of these coils is available with modern MRI machines, including dedicated coils for examination of the breast, neck and pelvis. These coils enable improved image quality by increasing the signal-to-noise ratio, but many have a limited field of view.

Contrast medium

Bowel opacification

- Bowel contrast media for use with MRI are now commercially available, but have not as yet gained widespread acceptance in clinical practice. A number of naturally occurring substances such as cranberry and pineapple juice have also proved effective as contrast agents. Oral contrast agents are of two types: those which produce delineation of the bowel by shortening T1 relaxation time (best evaluated on T1W images resulting in increased signal intensity - positive agents), and those which shorten T2/T2* relaxation time (best evaluated on T2/T2*-weighted sequences as negative agents).

Intravenous contrast medium

- IVCM may be given as an extracellular agent, e.g., Gadopentetate dimeglumine (also called Gadolinium-DTPA) or as an organ-specific agent, e.g., a liver-specific contrast agent. Extracellular IVCM for MRI is generally considered to be extremely safe, but some of the newer specific agents, e.g., iron containing compounds, may be associated with serious reactions and the supervising radiologist should be aware of these and their management.

Extracellular agents

- IVCM for opacification of vessels and for evaluation of the extravascular phase is an important component of many MRI examinations. The use of intravenous contrast medium should be planned according to examination protocols, but on occasion its use will be determined after review of the initial unenhanced sequences.

IV extracellular CM may be given as:

a) a rapid bolus injection combined with a rapid T1W dynamic scanning (gradient echo) technique (often using a mechanical injector), or

b) a bolus by hand injection followed by a routine non-dynamic T1W sequence.

The dose of intravenous contrast medium is usually 0.1 mmol/kg patient body weight although agents with higher relaxivity are usually given at lower doses.

Organ specific agents

The role of tissue-specific contrast agents continues to evolve.

- Liver-specific contrast agents are now commercially available and are broadly divided into two major groups: those which are taken up by the hepatocytes and those which are taken up by the reticuloendothelial system (i.e., super paramagnetic iron oxide or SPIO particles). Many studies have shown that liver enhancement using these agents is more sensitive in the detection of focal liver lesions than unenhanced MRI and such agents can also be used for lesion characterisation.

- Lymph node specific contrast agents for detection of metastases use ultrasmall super paramagnetic iron oxide particles (USPIO), which are taken up by the reticuloendothelial system. They are under investigation, but not yet commercially available.

Biopsy

Open magnetic systems which permit interventional techniques have been installed in a few centres in the United Kingdom. In general, biopsy under MRI guidance is a limited resource and, in most centres, biopsy continues to be undertaken under ultrasound or CT guidance. Specialised breast coils for breast biopsy are increasingly used. Special needles are available for biopsy of other regions.

Hard copy of CT and MR imaging

Multislice CT and MRI examinations produce a large number of images, particularly those examinations where dynamic scanning is employed. Review and reporting of the examination should be conducted on soft copy images at the diagnostic console. PACS systems are ideal for transferring image data for MDT meetings and other clinical uses. Robust systems of archival and retrieval of these large data files are required.

If PACS is not available, it is recommended that only sufficient images are printed to allow adequate presentation of the case in MDT meetings and for clinical colleagues to plan therapy.

Positron Emission Tomography (¹⁸FDG PET-CT)

PET and PET-CT using the commercially available radiotracer ¹⁸Fluoro-deoxyglucose (¹⁸FDG) identify the activity of cancer cells in masses demonstrated on CT and MR imaging and on occasion can detect functional abnormalities in structures which appear normal on CT and MR. Although ¹⁸FDG is not a truly tumour-specific agent, being a glucose ligand, clinical PET imaging using ¹⁸FDG is now becoming recognised as a key investigation for optimum management in several different malignancies. Depending on the tumour type, PET-CT can be a highly effective technique for primary tumour staging, assessing treatment response, as a prognostic indicator or for detecting disease recurrence. These applications of PET-CT have already been shown to alter patient management in approximately one third of patients with cancer. Current worldwide research is focusing on the development of tumour-specific radiotracers that can be detected by PET-CT scanners, for example, radiotracers linked to epidermal growth factor receptor (EGFR) or oestrogen receptor (ER) / HER-2 in breast cancer, and these developments coupled with further technological advances combining such state-of-the-art functional imaging with anatomical imaging (e.g., 64-slice PET-CT scanners and PET-MR scanners) will lead to an even more powerful modality in the years to come. Currently in the UK PET-CT is not yet widely available but a strategy for its implementation has been developed by the Department of Health and the Royal College of Radiologists.[11] The current document makes reference to the use of PET-CT in specific tumours where current evidence supports its use in routine clinical practice and its limitations in other tumours are also addressed in the appropriate disease sections.

Patient preparation

It is helpful for patients to receive general information about the scan prior to attendance in the department and this is best achieved in leaflet or booklet form. This should include a brief description of PET-CT scanning, the specific preparation that will be required, the time taken for the examination including waiting time in the department, and information about to whom and when the report will be sent.

Patient referrals are divided into two categories: those with insulin dependent diabetes (IDD), and all others. Patients with IDD are asked to drink plenty of water in the 6 hours leading up to the scan appointment (about 1 litre), but not too fast as it is unnecessary to disrupt blood glucose levels. All other patients are asked to abstain from food for at least 4 to 6 hours prior to the scan and also encouraged to drink plenty of water.

On arrival in the department, it is important to allow the patient an opportunity to ask questions so that he/she is as relaxed as possible, and for this reason appointment times should ideally include a pre-injection period of approximately 15 minutes. The patient should be comfortably warm prior to the scan because this will aid relaxation and reduce unwanted muscle and physiological brown fat uptake of ¹⁸FDG (a physiological normal variant which can be observed). It is important to diminish physiological uptake by brown fat because this can lead to errors in interpretation of the scan, particularly in the neck and axillae regions where nodal involvement from malignant melanoma, breast cancer, and head and neck cancers may also show uptake of ¹⁸FDG. In order to reduce physiological brown fat uptake, 5mg oral diazepam may be given one hour prior to the ¹⁸FDG injection. In addition to patients being staged for tumours which spread to the neck and axillae, the administration of diazepam is useful in young patients in whom ¹⁸FDG uptake by brown fat is common. Patients who are to be given diazepam should be escorted by a friend or relative.

Normal physiological muscle uptake of [18]FDG into the laryngeal muscles is demonstrated in patients who speak before, during or after tracer injection and this can cause confusion in interpretation of scans of the head and neck region. For this reason, it is recommended that patients with conditions involving the head and neck, e.g., head and neck cancer or lymphoma, observe a silence protocol with no speech for 20 minutes prior to the injection, during the injection period and for the majority of the uptake period (the first 30 minutes after injection being the most important period).

Injection site

It is critical that the member of staff performing the venepuncture and injection (usually the nuclear medicine technologist) is well trained and well practised as a precise technique is critical. Local extravasation results in a local radiation dose and can cause problems with scan interpretation, particularly as extravasated tracer is drained by the lymphatic system and therefore nodal uptake may be observed on the scan.

In patients with a history of carcinoma of the breast in particular, it is usually more appropriate to perform the tracer injection in the foot in order to avoid possible false positive axillary nodal uptake.

Patient positioning

Patients are routinely imaged with their arms raised above their head; this is important as it prevents beam hardening artefacts on the CT component of the study. Conversely, in patients with head and neck cancers, imaging is done with the arms down to their sides.

Radiation protection

With PET-CT, the radiation dose related to both the CT study and the PET tracers has to be taken into consideration for patients, technologists and the general public. The design and shielding of PET-CT imaging facilities may have to be modified appropriately and it is important to ensure that patients and staff are clear about all necessary precautions that should be undertaken. Radiation protection in relation to CT has already been discussed in this document (see CT section in this chapter); the remainder of this section addresses radiation protection issues related to the use of PET tracers.

It is important to remember that PET makes use of radiotracers with higher photon energy than those usually encountered in conventional nuclear medicine (511 keV compared to 140 keV). Furthermore, with faster imaging, the number of patients scanned daily will increase, as will the potential radiation exposure to staff, both to the whole body and to the extremities. Local legislation in the UK has set the annual whole-body dose limit for unclassified radiation workers at 6 mSv which is significantly lower than the previous limit of 15 mSv; this encumbers employers to ensure that staff are provided with all the means necessary to keep their doses below this level. These measures are detailed in the Royal College of Radiologists' 2005 publication *PET-CT in the UK: A strategy for development and integration of a leading edge technology within routine clinical practice.*[11]

The UK annual dose limit for members of the general public from medical sources is 1 mSv and there is a recommendation that at any one exposure, the dose should not exceed 30% of this.[12] Clearly, in a general waiting area there will not be just one PET patient, and an escort or carer could receive in excess of 0.3 mSv when taking into account the contribution from all the patients present. Ideally, it is best to have a "hot" waiting room separate from the "cold" waiting room, and the planning arrangements in the "hot" waiting room should ensure adequate separation of seating and preferably individually shielded cubicles for each patient. As the majority of PET scans will utilise [18]FDG, which has a very short half life, patients pose little risk to members of the public once they have completed their scans. The critical group where radiation exposure is likely to be higher is healthcare workers, who may have contact with several patients who have undergone PET investigations. Transport staff should be advised accordingly with specific instructions on the handling of body fluids. Current recommendations suggest that following an injected activity of 350 MBq of [18]FDG, there is no need to prevent contact with a patient's partner following a scan nor should there be restrictions on travel on public transport following the scan. However, some departments do advise patients to remain more than 1 metre away from others for about 10 hours after injection of the radiotracer. Clearly, young children should never accompany patients to the PET or nuclear medicine department and a patient's contact with them following injection of the radiotracer should also be avoided for about 10 hours.

Radiation dose

Combined PET-CT increases radiation exposure compared to CT or PET scans when performed alone. The radiation exposure from the CT component is considered to be lower than diagnostic CT, but is dependent on the exposure factors utilised for the measurement. Typically, when very low tube currents are used (30-50 mAs), the volume CT dose index ($CTDI_{vol}$) is 2-3.6 mGy; higher tube currents (e.g., 80 mAs) will incur greater radiation exposure (6-10 mGy). Readers should refer to the appendix where the national reference standards for $CTDI_{vol}$ for diagnostic scans are given.

The typical injected activity of [18]FDG for PET imaging is between 200-370 MBq and incurs a radiation exposure of between 5-9 mSv. When this is added to the radiation dose of the low dose CT for the same scan (e.g., 4-5 mSv for a 50 mAs scan and 8 mSv for an 80 mAs scan), the total dose can be computed to lie in the range of 17-20 mSv, although higher doses are reported in the literature (up to 25 mSV).[13] This compares to 14.5 ± 5 mSV derived from a recent survey on diagnostic (higher-dose) whole body, multislice CT examinations (excluding head and neck examinations).[14] These higher doses for PET-CT thus require medical justification of the radiation exposure and optimisation of the examination, both of which remain key elements of radiation protection for patients.

References

1.   Morcos SK. Acute serious and fatal reactions to contrast media: our current understanding. *Br J Radiol 2005*; 78: 686-93.

2.   *Making the Best Use of a Department of Clinical Radiology.* 5th Edition. Royal College of Radiologists, London, 2003; RCR Ref. No. BFCR(03)3.

3.   ICRP (2000). Managing patient dose in computed tomography. International Commission on Radiological Protection Publication 87. *Annals of the ICRP*, 30, No 4. Oxford, Pergamon.

4.   EC (1997). *European Commission Council Directive 97/43/EURATOM* of 30 June 1997 on health protection of individuals against the dangers of ionising radiation in relation to medical exposure. Off. J. Eur. Commun., L180: 22-27.

5.   IRMER (2000). *The Ionising Radiation (Medical Exposure) Regulations 2000.* SI (2000) No.1059. TSO, London.

6.   Keat N. CT scanner automatic exposure control systems. *MHRA Evaluation Report 05016*, Medicines and Healthcare Products Regulatory Agency, London, February 2005.

7. Shrimpton P C, Hillier M C, Lewis M A and Dunn M (2005). *Doses from computed tomography (CT) examinations in the UK – 2003 review.* Chilton, NRPB-W67. Available now from the website of the Health Protection Agency: http://www.hpa.org.uk/radiation/publications/w_series_reports/2005/nrpb_w67.htm.

8. Buls N, Pages J, De Mey J, Osteaux M. Evaluation of patient and staff doses during various CT fluoroscopy guided interventions. *Health Physics* 2003; 85: 165-173.

9. Paulson EK, Sheafor DH, Enterline DS et al. CT fluoroscopy-guided interventional procedures: techniques and radiation dose to radiologists. *Radiology* 2001; 220: 161-167.

10. Safe Sedation, Analgesia and Anaesthesia within the Radiology Department. Royal College of Radiologists, London, 2003; RCR Ref. No. BFCR(03)4. ISBN:1872599 91 5.

11. PET-CT in the UK: A strategy for development and integration of a leading edge technology within routine clinical practice. Royal College of Radiologists, London, 2005; RCR Ref. No. BRCR(05)5. ISBN:1 905034 05 9.

12. *Council Directive 96/29/Euratom of 13 May 1966 laying down basic safety standards for the protection of the health of workers and the general public against dangers arising from ionising radiation.* Official Journal of the European Communities: Council of the European Union; 1996. Report No.L159.

13. Brix G, Lechel U, Glatting G, et al. Radiation exposure of patients undergoing whole-body dual-modality 18F-FDG PET/CT examinations. *J Nucl Med* 2005; 46: 608-613.

14. Brix G, Nagel HD, Stamm G, et al. Radiation exposure in multi-slice versus single-slice spiral CT: results of a nationwide survey. *Eur Radiol 2003*; 13: 1979-1991.

24

CHAPTER 3

Lymph nodes

Clinical background

Staging of lymph nodes is an integral part of the TNM staging classification because nodal involvement is a powerful adverse prognostic indicator which often determines patient management, frequently distinguishing surgical candidates from those best suited to non-surgical management. In most cases the incidence of nodal involvement increases with tumour bulk and stage, and is dependent on histological type and grade. In order to provide the best possible assessment of the nodal status of patients, radiologists are required to:

a) Have detailed knowledge of tumour histology and stage of the primary tumour to determine the probability of nodal involvement (see Tips below).

b) Know of pattern of spread (see Tips below) and the prevalence of micro- as opposed to macroscopic nodal spread.

c) Be familiar with the criteria for nodal involvement on MRI/CT at various anatomical sites (see below), recognising pitfalls in diagnosis.

d) Have an idea of the accuracy of imaging observations and understand the impact of positive and negative imaging results on patient management.

e) Be familiar with new imaging methods for evaluating nodal disease.

The TNM system emphasises regional nodal involvement in the N category, but nodal involvement at other than regional sites is classified as distant metastases (i.e., belongs in the M category). It is therefore important for radiologists to know where regional and metastatic sites reside for each tumour site and these details can be found in staging manuals such as the AJCC *Cancer Staging Manual* (see chapter 1 for details). Sometimes, the same organ may have differing regional nodal groups; thus, the retroperitoneum is a metastatic site for cervical tumours but is defined as 'regional' for endometrial cancer.

The TNM emphasises different aspects for nodal involvement depending on the primary tumour; thus for the bladder and head and neck cancers, nodal size is part of the N category. For many adenocarcinomas, the presence or absence of microscopic metastatic disease, regardless of primary tumour burden, is emphasised whereas nodal involvement sometimes does not alter staging category at all (e.g., for well-differentiated follicular / papillary thyroid cancers in patients less than 45 years old).

Currently, the only widely available criterion for assessing lymph nodes by imaging techniques is nodal size assessed in the axial short-axis; nodal size criteria are set out in the table below. This assessment method is very limited in its accuracy, because it is unable to detect microscopic disease in normal size nodes (false negative result) and to distinguish enlarged, hyperplastic (benign) from malignant lymph nodes (false positive results). This limitation has important clinical implications for patients, for example those with lung cancer, where the only hope for cure is surgery and where operability is determined largely by the lymph node status in the mediastinum. As imaging has limited accuracy to stage mediastinal lymph nodes, patients with tumours that are considered potentially resectable often undergo another operation (mediastinoscopy with lymph node sampling) to pathologically assess the lymph nodes before definitive resection is performed. This situation has improved with the more widespread introduction of ^{18}FDG PET-CT scanning and the expected imminent introduction of MR lymphography using USPIO contrast medium (see chapter 2 for more details).

Who should be imaged?

All patients undergoing staging investigations that involve imaging for diagnosed or suspected cancer should have nodal status assessed.

Staging objectives

- To identify presence / extent of regional nodal metastases with a view to assigning an N-staging category.

- To identify whether the extent of nodal disease will significantly alter the surgical approach. For example, by increasing the extent of surgical exploration required for the placement of vascular grafts.

- To determine whether the presence of metastatic nodal involvement designates M-stage disease.

- To identify presence / extent of regional nodal enlargement with a view to planning biopsy.

- To distinguish between nodal enlargement due to malignancy and that due to benign hyperplasia.

- To attempt to detect the presence of microscopic disease in normal size nodes (only currently possible with MR lymphography and ^{18}FDG PET-CT).

Staging

Nodal assessment forms part of the TNM assessment and should be undertaken using CT or MRI, as appropriate, using nodal size criteria as defined below. The areas to be examined are as appropriate for the primary tumour.

Staging the primary tumour should be undertaken according to the guidelines in this document.

Lymph node size at various anatomic sites: short axis diameter, upper limits of normal		
Site	Group	Short axis size (mm)
Head and Neck [1]	Facial Cervical	Not visible 10 (<10 mm with central necrosis)
Axilla		10
Mediastinum [3,4,5]	Subcarinal Paracardiac Retrocrural All other sites	12 8 6 10
Abdomen [5]	Gastrohepatic ligament Porta hepatis Portacaval Coeliac axis to renal artery Renal artery to aortic bifurcation	8 8 10 10 12
Pelvis [6]	Common iliac External iliac Internal iliac Obturator	9 10 7 8
Inguinal		10

Follow-up

As appropriate for individual tumour sites.

Tips

- Morphological criteria that can be useful for nodal assessment include:
  - Nodal size (see above).
  - Nodal shape (round or elliptical).
  - Nodal contour (to identify extracapsular spread).
  - Nodal clustering.
  - Nodal density (particularly cystic or necrotic regions).
  - Enhancement characteristics following intravenous contrast medium administration (homogeneity / heterogeneity / central necrosis).

- Although not required for the TNM staging, it is sometimes necessary to classify in detail the sites of regional nodal involvement in order to facilitate surgical exploration (e.g., for head and neck tumours and in lung cancer – see relevant chapters for details).

- There is often confusion about the precise anatomical location of nodal sites on cross-sectional imaging, particularly when planning radiotherapy. It is recommended that a standard nodal atlas is used (e.g., Martinez-Monge 1999).[7]

- Assessment of the probability of nodal involvement according to the histology, clinical extent and serum tumour marker levels for a number of different tumours can be found in the literature for some tumours (e.g., breast, prostate, and renal). These prediction tools can sometimes help radiologists make a reasonable assumption when evaluating individual patients and can be found at nomograms@mskcc.org

- It must be remembered that ^{18}FDG PET-CT and MR lymphography with USPIO contrast enhancement do not provide the same information and may not be equally efficacious (no direct comparisons appear in the literature); thus, the sensitivity of ^{18}FDG PET-CT is dependent on tumour type (e.g., less sensitive in prostate cancer), tumour biology in terms of rate of growth (less efficacious in non-seminomatous germ cell tumours), on histological type (less good for evaluating alveolar cell or colloidal neoplasms) and other factors. However, in several tumour types ^{18}FDG PET-CT is an accurate modality for detecting nodal involvement. Depending on the tumour type, nodes less than 10 mm in size can be identified.

References:

1. Tart RP, Mukherji SK, Avino AJ, et al. Facial lymph nodes: normal and abnormal CT appearance. *Radiology* 1993; 188: 695-700.

2. van der Brekel MWM, Stel HV, Castelijns JA, et al. Cervical lymph node metastasis: assessment of radiological criteria. *Radiology* 1990; 177: 379-384.

3. Glazer GM, Gross BH, Quint LE, et al. Normal mediastinal lymph nodes: number and size according to American Thoracic Society mapping. *AJR Am J Roentgenol* 1985; 144: 261-265.

4. Dorfman RE, Alpern MB, Gross BH, Sandler MA. Upper abdominal lymph nodes: criteria for normal size determined with CT. *Radiology* 1991; 180: 319-322.

5. Callen PW, Korobkin M, Isherwood I. Computed tomography evaluation of the retrocrural, prevertebral space. *AJR Am J Roentgenol* 1977; 129: 907-910.

6. Vinnicombe S, Norman A, Husband JE, Nicolson V. Normal pelvic lymph nodes: documentation by CT scanning after bipedal lymphangiography. *Radiology* 1995; 194: 349-355.

7. Martinez-Monge R, Fernandes PS, Gupta N, Gahbauer R. Cross-sectional nodal atlas: a tool for the definition of clinical target volumes in three-dimensional radiation therapy planning. *Radiology* 1999; 211(3): 815-828.

CHAPTER 4

Tumours of the brain

Brain primary tumours

Clinical background

Attempts at developing a TNM-based classification and staging system for central nervous system tumours have been unsuccessful because of poor compliance and the lack of utility in predicting patient outcome. Reasons for this include the fact that primary tumour (T-stage) size is significantly less relevant than tumour histology and location in predicting outcome. Nodal staging (N-stage) does not apply to brain tumours, and metastases (M-stage), when they do occur, are usually found in paediatric neoplasms and spread is through the cerebrospinal fluid.

Who should be imaged?

All patients suspected of having a primary brain tumour should be imaged initially with MRI or CT.

Imaging objectives

- To detect tumour.

- To characterise tumour.

- To determine extent of tumour.

- To select optimal site for obtaining histological material (preferably where tumour grade is highest and avoiding eloquent areas and those with a large amount of necrosis or of cyst formation).

MRI is the investigation of choice in the evaluation of primary cerebral neoplasms. It is superior to CT for tumour detection due to better contrast resolution, which gives a high sensitivity to any alteration in the nature of brain tissue. However, CT can provide unique information not readily available on MRI (e.g., the presence of calcification) and is still used in the primary investigation of non-specific neurological presentations, which may occasionally be caused by the tumour. If a mass-like lesion is detected on CT, MRI should be undertaken for further characterisation and to assess the full extent of disease. Nevertheless, MRI is unable to predict tumour type and histological grade reliably. Signal intensity and contrast enhancement characteristics may assist the surgeon in choosing a site for biopsy and imaging may be used for guiding stereotactic biopsy procedures. Proton MR Spectroscopy (^{1}H-MRS), single photon emission computed tomography (SPECT) and positron emission tomography (PET) remain experimental procedures in the evaluation of brain tumours. High resolution CT is useful in addition to MRI in pre-operative assessment and follow-up of skull base tumours.

Imaging should be able to discriminate between tumours and other intracranial mass lesions, e.g., infarcts, haemorrhage or inflammatory / demyelinating lesions. Some tumours have characteristic features on imaging which allow a definite diagnosis to be reached prior to biopsy. However, most tumours will need to be biopsied for histological classification.

Unlike tumours elsewhere in the body, a biopsy is not usually obtained prior to definitive surgery. Intra-operative histological evaluation by a specialist neuropathologist is, however, commonly obtained. A decision will be made on imaging as to whether image-guided biopsy, open biopsy or resection is most appropriate for patient management. In some instances, it will be decided that biopsy is neither feasible nor clinically appropriate. Depending on the presumed diagnosis, these patients may have surveillance follow-up imaging or referral for palliative radiotherapy.

Imaging

MRI

For the majority of supratentorial tumours conventional MR imaging is undertaken with the use of intravenous contrast medium enhancement using a small molecular weight, extracellular gadolinium containing contrast agent such as Gd-DTPA. As 70% of adult brain tumours are supratentorial the following technique is advised.

Protocol for imaging of adult brain tumours			
Sequence	Plane	Slice thickness	Field of view
T2W	Axial	6 ± 1 mm	Whole brain
FLAIR*	Axial + Coronal	6 ± 1 mm	Whole brain
T1W	Coronal / Axial	6 ± 1 mm	Whole brain
T1W with contrast medium enhancement	Axial / Coronal	6 ± 1 mm	Whole brain

*Fluid attenuated inversion recovery

Surgeons usually like at least one sequence in the sagittal plane in addition to the above to aid in surgical planning. Diffusion-weighted imaging (DWI) is of value in discriminating between infarcts and tumours, and abscesses and necrotic or cystic tumours.

Variations to the standard "brain" protocol are necessary for investigation of parasellar tumours and tumours of the cerebellopontine angle, such as acoustic schwannomas.

In the paediatric population, a higher percentage of tumours (around 50%) are located in the posterior fossa. Sagittal imaging can be useful in assessment of medulloblastoma and other midline tumours, such as pineoblastomas and germ cell tumours which tend to occur in younger patients.

Pre-operative MRI of the whole spine to look for meningeal "drop" metastases is essential in paediatric patients with tumours of the posterior fossa or pineal gland.

Protocol for imaging the spine for meningeal metastases			
Sequence	Plane	Slice thickness	Field of view
T1 pre- and post-contrast medium	Sagittal	3 ± 1 mm	Large
T1 pre- and post-contrast medium	Axial where abnormal	4 ± 1 mm	Small

CT

- 1-5 mm axial sections using spiral technique from the skull base to the vertex, parallel to the clivus to avoid irradiation of the orbits.

- Scans should be obtained pre- and post-injection of 50-100 ml of intravenous contrast medium.

- Using MDCT, slice thickness will depend on scanner capability. In general, sections are acquired at 1.25-2.5 mm and reformatted at 5 mm for viewing.

Values of $CTDI_{vol}$ should normally be below the relevant national reference dose for the region of scan and patient group (see Appendix and section on *Radiation Protection for the Patient in CT* in chapter 2).

Immediate pre- and intra-operative imaging

Both CT and MRI are used for directing image-guided biopsy. This will be performed in dedicated neurosurgical units. Additional sequences that aid in surgical planning may need to be performed. These will include DWI, MR angiography (MRA), MR venography (MRV) and CT angiography (CTA). MRS, SPECT and PET are all techniques that may be of value in identifying the area of highest grade of malignancy and therefore influence choice of biopsy site.

Follow-up

Patients may be treated by complete or partial resection, radiotherapy, chemotherapy or by adopting a wait and watch policy. The requirement for follow-up imaging of different CNS tumours is variable and the Neuroscience and Cancer Network MDT will usually determine follow-up protocols.

In obtaining any follow-up imaging, care should be taken to obtain sequences in an identical manner to previous investigations, including the same scanning plane (including angle), slice thickness and sequence type. When hard copy rather than PACS is used for archiving imaging data, it is advisable to have an agreed convention with the local Neuroscience Unit for displaying images in terms of orientation (e.g., sagittal, right to left; coronal, front to back; axial, bottom to top). This allows for ease of comparison on subsequent follow-up imaging.

Following surgery, meningeal enhancement is frequently seen and may last for years. Enhancement of the parenchyma adjacent to the resection cavity usually appears within the first 24 hours but resolves in 6-12 months. It is seen earlier and more clearly on MR imaging than on CT. A variety of changes, including white matter signal abnormality, may be seen following radiotherapy. Since the incidence of recurrence of brain tumours is high, it is useful to have a post-treatment baseline scan approximately 3 months after completion of therapy. Further imaging is indicated when new symptoms develop. Paediatric tumours are commonly scanned within 24 hours of surgery to assess the extent of residual disease.

Follow-up of *gliomas* is variable and depends on the underlying histology, patient symptoms and the nature and extent of treatment undertaken. Prolonged survival with low-grade glioma is common, but these tumours may transform to high-grade glioma. Imaging at follow-up should use the same protocols as at diagnosis. Follow-up scans are performed at intervals as determined by the local MDT.

Acoustic neuromas and pituitary tumours are other examples of tumours which may require long-term imaging follow-up.

Protocol for imaging of acoustic neuroma			
Sequence	Plane	Slice thickness	Field of view
T2W	Axial / Coronal	6 ± 1 mm	Whole brain
T2W	Axial / Coronal	3 ± 0.3 mm	Small
T1W	Axial	3 ± 0.3 mm	Small
T1W with contrast medium enhancement	Axial	3 ± 0.3 mm	Small

When screening for possible acoustic neuroma, 3-D volume T2W sequences such as CISS (contiguous imaging steady state) or DRIVE (driven equilibrium radio frequency reset pulse) are usually sufficient.

Acoustic neuromas are commonly managed with surveillance scanning. Volume T2W using the sequences described above is usually sufficient, but post-contrast T1 in the axial and coronal planes may be performed. Post-operative follow-up of acoustic neuromas does require a contrast medium enhanced scan to detect nodular areas of recurrence. Linear enhancement of the internal auditory meatus (IAM) and adjacent dura is a normal post-surgical finding.

Protocol for imaging of pituitary or parasellar tumours			
Sequence	Plane	Slice thickness	Field of view
T2W / FLAIR	Axial	6 ± 1 mm	Whole brain
T1W	Sagittal & Coronal	3 ± 0.3 mm	Small
T2W	Coronal	3 ± 0.3 mm	Small

Enhancement with gadolinium is not recommended for routine use in the investigation of pituitary microadenoma. In Cushing's, growth hormone deficiency or diabetes insipidus contrast medium enhancement is required. On the first examination of a presumed pituitary macroadenoma, contrast medium enhancement will be helpful to discriminate between other sellar or suprasellar tumours, e.g., craniopharyngiomas or meningiomas.

Follow-up imaging of histologically verified pituitary macroadenomas does not normally require contrast medium enhancement. A baseline scan should be obtained at 4-6 months post-surgery, as reduction in size of any residual soft tissue within the sella occurs during that time.

Tips

- The TNM system is not useful for primary brain tumours.
- Histology of tumour is by far the most important prognostic factor.
- MRI should be able to discriminate between tumours and other intracranial lesions.

- Following treatment, meningeal enhancement may be prolonged and should be interpreted with caution.
- Pre-contrast CT may demonstrate calcification and haemorrhage frequently obscured on post-contrast scans.

Brain metastases

Clinical background

All malignant tumours can metastasise to brain with lung, breast and melanoma doing so most frequently. Brain metastases from gastrointestinal (GI) and genitourinary tract (GU) tumours occur less commonly. The majority of metastases (80%) are supratentorial; however, GI and GU tumour metastases are more common in the posterior fossa, 50% being infratentorial. Within the cerebral hemispheres the grey / white matter junction is the most common site of metastases. Diagnosis is usually made on the basis of multiple lesions, but solitary brain metastases occur and may be resectable. Multiple lesions are treated with chemotherapy which will include the use of corticosteroids or radiotherapy, which may be to whole brain or to individual lesions (stereotactic external beam radiotherapy or gamma knife irradiation). Metastases are usually of high signal intensity on T2W imaging and of intermediate signal intensity on T1W imaging, although this signal pattern is sometimes reversed in haemorrhagic metastases, melanoma and mucinous adenocarcinoma. There is usually surrounding oedema and the degree may be variable, but it is often disproportionate to the size of the lesion. Metastases situated in the grey matter tend to be associated with less oedema than those found in the white matter. Enhancement with contrast medium is typical and may be seen throughout the lesion or only at its rim.

Meningeal metastatic disease is diagnosed by the presence of multiple enhancing nodules in the leptomeninges. Dural enhancement may be normal within the cranial cavity particularly after a CSF tap. Meningeal metastatic disease may be present in the absence of meningeal enhancement and confirmed by cytology even when MRI is entirely normal. Conversely, no malignant cells may be found on cytology despite abnormal meningeal enhancement.

Who should be imaged?

All patients with a previous history of malignancy and symptoms or signs suggesting metastatic disease to the brain should be imaged initially with MRI or CT.

Imaging objectives

- To detect the presence of brain metastases.
- To identify the number of metastases.
- To determine tumour extent.

Imaging

MRI

Protocol for imaging of brain metastases			
Sequence	Plane	Slice thickness	Field of view
T2W	Axial	6 ± 1 mm	Whole brain
FLAIR	Axial	6 ± 1 mm	Whole brain
T1W	Axial	6 ± 1 mm	Whole brain
T1W with contrast medium	Axial / Coronal	6 ± 1 mm	Whole brain

The dose of gadolinium containing contrast medium given may vary with therapeutic intent. Normally, 0.1 mmol/kg patient body weight of Gd-DTPA is given (or equivalent, if contrast agents of higher relaxivity are used), but this may be increased to increase the sensitivity. Higher doses may be used if resection or targeted irradiation is being contemplated.

CT

- 1-5 mm axial sections using spiral technique from the skull base to the vertex, parallel to the clivus to avoid irradiation of the orbits.
- Scans should be obtained pre- and post-injection of 50-100 ml of intravenous contrast medium.
- Using MDCT, slice thickness will depend on scanner capability. In general, sections are acquired at 1.25-2.5 mm and reformatted at 5 mm for viewing.

Values of $CTDI_{vol}$ should normally be below the relevant national reference dose for the region of scan and patient group (see Appendix and section on *Radiation Protection for the Patient in CT* in chapter 2).

PET-CT

Although intracranial metastases may show uptake with [18]FDG, PET-CT is not generally used for intracranial lesion detection because grey matter demonstrates (normal) physiological uptake of this tracer.

Follow-up

After resection / targeted radiotherapy of a solitary metastasis or whole brain radiotherapy for multiple brain metastases, follow-up MRI may be performed 3 months after completion of treatment to serve as a baseline. However, patients may also be managed expectantly and only re-imaged when new symptoms develop. Again, the imaging technique should be the same as that used at diagnosis of metastatic disease.

CT is sometimes used at diagnosis and follow-up. If a firm diagnosis of multiple metastases can be made by the presence of enhancing lesions in the brain and treatment can be planned accordingly, it may not be necessary to undertake MRI at follow-up. However, contrast-enhanced MRI is the most accurate available technique for establishing the site, size and number of metastatic intracranial lesions and is best for the follow-up also.

Tips

- Pre-contrast CT or MRI scans are useful in patients with suspected metastases from testicular non-seminomatous germ cell tumours which are frequently haemorrhagic.
- Malignant melanoma metastases are frequently of high signal intensity on pre-contrast MRI T1W images due to the paramagnetic effects of melanin, and of high density on pre-contrast CT scans.

CHAPTER 5

Tumours of the spinal cord

Primary spinal cord tumours

Clinical background

Primary spinal cord tumours are relatively rare, accounting for approximately 1% of all CNS tumours. Clinical features will usually indicate the level of involvement in the spinal cord. Low-grade gliomas and ependymomas account for the majority of primary spinal cord tumours.

Who should be imaged?

All patients with symptoms and signs suggesting a primary spinal cord tumour should be investigated initially with MRI.

Imaging objectives

- MRI is the investigation of choice in all patients with suspected spinal cord tumours.
- The objective is to define presence and extent of tumour and suitability for surgery.
- The region of the primary tumour should be examined in detail.
- The whole spinal cord and cauda equina should be imaged, as these lesions may be extensive and diffuse. Ependymomas may metastasise throughout the subarachnoid space.

Imaging

MRI

When a lesion has been identified in the thoracic spine or spinal cord, it is essential that a sagittal T2W scan, which demonstrates the level of the lesion in relationship to the lumbar sacral junction, is obtained. This enables the surgeon to identify the level for the laminectomy using x-ray fluoroscopy in the operating theatre.

Protocol for imaging of primary spinal cord neoplasms			
Sequence	Plane	Slice thickness	Field of view
T1W	Sagittal	4 ± 1 mm	Large
T2W	Sagittall	4 ± 1 mm	Large
T1W with contrast medium enhancement	Sagittal	4 ± 1 mm	Large
T2W or T1W with contrast medium	Axial	5 ± 2 mm	Small

Follow-up

A post-treatment baseline scan 3 months after surgery or radiotherapy is useful and further imaging may be obtained as determined by symptoms or as protocolled by the MDT.

Tip

- The majority of primary spinal cord tumours are of low histological grade.

Metastatic spinal cord tumours

Clinical background

Metastases may involve the spinal meninges and the intra-axial cord. Common solid tumours such as breast, lung and melanoma will metastasise to the meninges by haematogenous spread, but this tends to occur late in the natural history of the disease usually in the presence of metastatic disease at other sites. Primary tumours of the CNS may also metastasise to the meninges by spread through the CSF. These include glioblastoma, pineal tumours, choroid plexus papilloma / carcinoma, and especially posterior fossa tumours of childhood such as primitive neuroectodermal tumours (PNET) and ependymomas.

Symptoms may be complex and not localised to a single anatomical site. A poorly localised headache or backache may be present. It is important to identify patients who may have meningeal metastatic disease because this significantly alters imaging technique. Gadolinium contaminating contrast medium enhancement is obligatory to increase the sensitivity of MRI for the detection of meningeal disease.

Who should be imaged?

All patients with neurological deficit or persistent symptoms suggestive of metastases to the spinal meninges or intra-axial spinal cord.

Imaging objectives

- To identify the presence, location, extent and number of spinal cord metastases.
- To identify meningeal involvement.

Imaging

MRI

The whole spine must be imaged. Axial T1W gadolinium enhanced images may also be obtained to define lesion location. Intra-axial spinal cord disease presents clinically in a similar way to meningeal metastatic disease, and the imaging technique is the same.

Sequence	Plane	Slice thickness	Field of view
T2W	Sagittal	4 ± 1 mm	Large
T1W	Sagittall	4 ± 1 mm	Large
T1W with contrast medium	Sagittal	4 ± 1 mm	Large

Follow-up

A post-treatment baseline scan 3 months after surgery or radiotherapy is useful and further imaging may be obtained as determined by symptoms or as protocolled by the MDT.

Tips

- Meningeal metastatic disease from solid tumours tends to occur late in the natural history of the disease.

- If intra-axial spinal cord deposits or meningeal metastatic disease is considered a clinical possibility, gadolinium enhancement is required for an adequate MRI study.

Spinal cord compression

Clinical background

Metastatic bone disease to the bony spine is capable of compressing the spinal cord. Impending cord compression is one of the few indications for emergency imaging in oncological practice. The principal clinical features include pain, power loss, sensory disturbance and impaired sphincter function. While power loss is progressing, there is a chance of regaining function. Steroids should be started, and MR imaging undertaken within 24 hours. Sphincter disturbance requires more urgent imaging, because delay can lead to non-reversible functional loss. Referral to a neurosurgical centre may be indicated, and radiotherapy can be planned while waiting for imaging to confirm level(s) of compression. Primary bone tumours or soft tissue masses such as lymphoma, neuroblastoma, neurofibromas or meningiomas may also cause compression of the spinal cord.

Who should be imaged?

All patients with symptoms and signs of spinal cord compression should be referred for MRI, which may be undertaken at a neurosurgical centre or at a general hospital.

Imaging objectives

- To determine the presence, extent, and level of spinal cord compression.

- To identify multiple sites of spinal cord compression.

- To identify sites of incipient spinal cord compression elsewhere in the spinal canal.

- To determine whether surgery is indicated.

- To detect the presence of soft tissue tumour.

Imaging

MRI

MRI is the investigation of choice, although CT may be useful in detecting paravertebral mass lesions.

Protocol for imaging spinal cord compression			
Sequence	Plane	Slice thickness	Field of view
T2W	Sagittal	4 ± 1 mm	Large
T1W	Sagittall	4 ± 1 mm	Medium
T2W	Axial	3.5 ± 1 mm	Small

The entire spine must always be imaged in suspected cord compression as multiple levels may be detected. Sagittal imaging, which shows the relationship of the lesion to the lumbar sacral junction, must be included to allow planning for surgery or radiotherapy. When there is doubt about a transitional lumbosacral junction then the craniocervical junction must be adequately demonstrated.

If pain restricts the number of sequences which can be performed, T1W imaging of the whole spine should be completed before any further investigation. This is a highly specific for metastatic disease. Standard T2W imaging gives a better myelographic effect and thus improves delineation of the extent of cord compression which maybe side-to-side due to involvement of vertebral pedicles. Occasionally, it is necessary to use a STIR sequence in the sagittal plane which is a sensitive method for detecting lytic metastatic disease but performs poorly for delineating the extent of cord compression owing to blurring from motion artefacts. Gradient-echo T2*W sequences and contrast medium enhancement are occasionally helpful for differentiating acute osteoporotic vertebral fractures from metastatic causes of vertebral collapse.

CT

CT and CT myelography have little place in imaging of spinal cord pathology but are still required on occasion in patients where MRI is contra-indicated or not obtainable in the emergency setting. CT imaging may also provide information on integrity of bone prior to surgical spinal stabilisation.

Values of $CTDI_{vol}$ should normally be below the relevant national reference dose for the region of scan and patient group (see Appendix and section on *Radiation Protection for the Patient in CT* in chapter 2).

Follow-up

A post-treatment baseline scan 3 months after surgery or radiotherapy is useful and further imaging may be obtained as determined by symptoms or as protocolled by the MDT.

Tip

- In a patient with known malignancy and clinical evidence of spinal cord compression, the entire spine should be imaged.

CHAPTER 6

Head & neck cancers

Introduction

Cancers of the head and neck mostly arise from the mucosal surfaces of the upper aerodigestive tract (most are thus squamous cell tumours). The T-staging which indicates the extent of the primary tumour is generally similar but differs in specific details related to the anatomical site of the primary tumour. In general, the N-classification is uniform for all anatomical sites except for nasopharynx and thyroid because of differing tumour biology and prognosis. The status of regional lymph nodes provides such important prognostic information that nodes should be assessed in detail in terms of location, multiplicity, size, neurovascular involvement and extranodal tumour spread. Not only is it important to note whether upper or lower neck lymph nodes are involved (the dividing line is the lower border of the cricoid) but it is important that specific anatomical subsites are included / excluded as being involved. As far as possible, neck nodal sites should be identified by nature and level to facilitate understanding between the radiologist and the clinician of sites of disease (e.g., submental [level 1A], upper deep cervical [level 2], etc.). These nodal levels conform to surgical landmarks identified at the time of surgical neck exploration. The natural history and response to therapy of metastatic nodal disease from the nasopharynx differs from tumours arising from other mucosal sites which require a different N-classification. Similarly, nodal involvement in well-differentiated thyroid cancer does not significantly alter patient prognosis and thus a unique N-staging has been developed.

[18]FDG PET is an effective technique for imaging head and neck cancer. It has a higher sensitivity than CT for detecting lesions due to the difficulty of visualising small soft tissue tumours within the complex anatomy of the region. [18]FDG PET also has a high specificity. Where available, it should be used as an adjunct to CT and MRI staging, providing more accurate information in assessing primary tumour extent as well as metastatic nodal disease in the neck. A significantly high proportion of occult primary tumours may be detected by PET-CT. The majority of these are in the region of the base of the tongue (MRI and CT not being sensitive with regard to small tongue tumours). [18]FDG PET-CT has a major advantage over anatomical imaging in the assessment of the neck following surgery / radiotherapy, being able to detect and accurately re-stage disease recurrence.

Nasopharynx

Clinical background

Cancer of the nasopharynx is peculiar in having a unique geographical distribution (Southern China) and consistently high levels of Ebstein-Barr virus antibodies. When nasopharyngeal cancers occur in Europeans, smoking and sawmill dust are additional causative factors. Squamous cell carcinoma is the commonest nasopharyngeal malignancy and most of these tumours present late, often with lymph node metastases which can be bilateral. Tumours usually arise in the Fossa of Rosenmuller and often spread submucosally and deeply. Distant metastases occur at presentation in less than 10% of cases, with lung, bone and liver being the most common sites of spread. The incidence of distant spread of disease in nasopharyngeal cancer is higher than with other head and neck tumours; rates of 30-50% are reported for N3 disease (i.e., metastasis in a lymph node greater than 6 cm in size and/or supraclavicular nodal enlargement). Many cases are detected on routine scanning for non-specific nasal or otalgic symptoms. Radiotherapy is the mainstay of treatment and imaging is designed to evaluate patients for this.

Who should be imaged?

MRI is indicated in all patients with biopsy-proven nasopharyngeal cancer. CT is often performed as the initial investigation for non-specific sino-nasal symptoms. If this demonstrates advanced disease, no further imaging is required.

The aim of imaging is to document local extent of tumour, particularly erosion into the skull base, and the presence and extent of nodal metastases. The stage of the disease can significantly alter the choice of radiotherapy technique used. The TNM staging system has been modified to take account of the additional information now available from MRI scanning, and it should be noted that CT generally overstages nasopharynx cancer compared to MRI. MRI is the imaging modality of choice for staging, particularly for perineural spread and skull base invasion. In clinically advanced disease at presentation, CT may be adequate to assess the primary tumour and extent of nodal spread.

Staging objectives

- To identify extent of local tumour.
- To identify extent and distribution of lymph node metastases.
- To identify organs at risk for radiotherapy damage.

Staging

MRI

T-staging is best achieved with imaging in multiple planes. Contrast enhancement, with gadolinium containing chelates with or without fat suppression, is recommended for demonstration of perineural spread. A combination of axial, coronal and sagittal imaging is usually required for full assessment and treatment planning. MRI is as accurate as CT for N-staging of the neck. The area from the skull base (top of clinoids) down to supraclavicular fossa should be included in the examination.

Protocol for imaging of acoustic neuroma				
Sequence	Plane	Slice thickness	Field of view	Reason
STIR T1W T2W Fat Sat T1W	Coronal Coronal Axial Axial	3 mm (max) 3 mm 3 mm 5-6 mm	Small Small Small Small	Identification of primary tumour and survey of neck for nodes
T1W + Gad Fat Sat	Axial	5-6 mm	Small	To look for perineural spread
T1W + Gad Fat Sat	Coronal	3 mm	Small	To look for perineural spread Assess intracranial extension
T1 + Gad Fat Sat	Sagittal	3 mm	Small	Aid to Radiotherapy Planning

CT

CT is not as accurate as MRI for assessing the soft tissue extent of the tumour (T-staging) but is important for detecting bone involvement.

- 3 mm axial sections using spiral technique, following intravenous contrast enhancement, through skull base.

- 5 mm axial sections using spiral technique through the neck.

- Using MDCT, slice thickness will depend on scanner capability. In general, sections are acquired at 1.25-2.5 mm and reformatted no greater than 3-5 mm for viewing.

Values of $CTDI_{vol}$ should normally be below the relevant national reference dose for the region of scan and patient group (see Appendix and section on *Radiation Protection for the Patient* in CT in chapter 2).

PET-CT

[18]FDG PET-CT is a useful technique for the detection and re-staging of post-treatment disease recurrence

Follow-up

Reassessment imaging is often performed 3 months following completion of radiotherapy. It is advisable to use the same technique employed for initial staging at follow-up. Further imaging follow-up usually then depends on disease status and clinical symptoms.

Tips

- Imaging head and neck tumours in general does not determine the decision to treat the neck nodes – this is based on the primary tumour site and the pathology.

- The nasopharynx does not usually revert to normal following radiotherapy. Residual soft tissue effacement is generally seen even after successful treatment.

Larynx

Clinical background

This is the commonest head & neck cancer site. Significant imaging developments have improved our ability to detect deep spread that may be clinically occult. Patterns of spread can alter the treatment strategy which is usually either surgery or radiotherapy. Separate primary site classification systems are used for supraglottic, glottic, and subglottic tumours. Vocal cord fixation upstages all tumours to T3 classification. Cartilage invasion is often clinically occult but upstages tumours to T4. Imaging is more accurate than clinical staging and has a major role in the assessment of potential larynx-preserving surgery techniques. Surgery or radiotherapy may be used as the primary treatment depending on the stage of disease. Cartilage invasion is generally considered an indication for more radical surgery.

The lymphatic drainage of the larynx is complex. It depends on the site of the tumour and the depth of invasion. The glottis has a very sparse lymphatic network whereas the supraglottic and subglottic larynx both have very rich lymphatic networks. Contralateral nodal involvement is common but it should be noted that midline nodal disease is considered unilateral.

Who should be imaged?

The diagnosis of larynx cancer is made on laryngoscopy. The contribution of imaging is to complement endoscopy by assessing the cartilages, the subglottic space and the tongue base, in particular.

Cross-sectional imaging is recommended for T2 lesions or above. Lower stage tumours may not be detectable on imaging, but imaging may be indicated where clinical assessment is difficult, or early subglottic disease is suspected.

CT is generally preferred as the imaging technique of choice because of speed of acquisition and patient tolerance. MRI is the best technique for assessing pre-epiglottic space and tongue base invasion. MRI is effective at demonstrating intracartilagenous tumour spread.

Staging objectives

- To identify extent of local tumour.
- To identify extent and distribution of lymph node metastases.
- To identify evidence of cartilage invasion.

Staging

CT

- 1-2 mm axial sections from hard palate, parallel to inferior border of mandible, down to thoracic inlet with intravenous contrast medium injection. Arms down by the patient's side. Instruct patient not to swallow during data acquisition which lasts only a few seconds.

- Using MDCT, slice thickness will depend on scanner capability. In general, sections are acquired at 0.625-1.25 mm and reformatted no greater than at 2.5 mm for viewing.

- CT of the thorax is indicated for disease clinically suspected to be Stage T2.

Values of CTDI$_{vol}$ should normally be below the relevant national reference dose for the region of scan and patient group (see Appendix and section on *Radiation Protection for the Patient in CT* in chapter 2).

MRI

MRI is useful in specific situations such as assessing possible pre-epiglottic space and tongue base invasion, and possible early cartilage invasion. Degraded images from swallowing motion artefacts are a problem that occurs particularly in patients whose airway is compromised by tumour. A combination of axial, sagittal and coronal T1W and T2W sequences may be required to assess the region of the larynx in question. Contrast medium enhancement with spectral fat suppression is useful for evaluating the extent of soft tissue involvement.

PET-CT

Physiological uptake of [18]FDG is observed in the larynx due to vocal cord activity. Therefore, a 'silence' protocol is required prior to performing PET-CT studies (i.e., the patient remaining silent for an hour prior to the study; see chapter 2 for further details). [18]FDG PET-CT can be useful to detect and define the extent of submucosal spread of disease.

Follow-up

Imaging 3-4 months after completion of radiotherapy is useful in documenting tumour response and serves as a baseline for future comparisons. The same imaging technique should be used as for the pre-treatment evaluation.

Tips

- Swallowing artefact and cord palsy can both mimic tumour. Repeating the study immediately is possible without the need for further contrast administration if it is apparent that the images are degraded by swallowing artefact.

- It is essential to scan the larynx in the correct plane to avoid misinterpretation.

Paranasal sinuses

Clinical background

Tumours of the paranasal sinuses are the least common (3-4%) of all head and neck malignancies. They are often advanced tumours at presentation and hence have a generally poor prognosis. Early disease often presents clinically as infection and may well have co-existent inflammatory change visible on imaging. The majority (80%) are squamous cell tumours and the maxillary antra are commonest sites of involvement. Other tumour histologies suggest minor salivary gland origin. Tumour spread is by direct infiltration and by perineural extension. Bone destruction is common. In contrast to other head & neck tumours, lymph node spread is uncommon. Distant spread is also uncommon (10%) and when present involves spread to the lungs and bones. Treatment for paranasal sinus tumours is usually a combination of primary surgery and adjuvant radiotherapy. The main cause of treatment failure is local recurrence.

Who should be imaged?

Imaging is indicated in all patients with biopsy proven paranasal sinus cancer. A combination of CT and MRI is generally required for complete staging prior to treatment. CT is often performed as the initial investigation for non-specific symptoms. If advanced disease is demonstrated, which is not appropriate for surgical management, no further imaging is required.

The role of imaging is to help plan the surgical approach and to define the radiation fields subsequently. The anatomy is complex and interactive review of imaging in MDT meetings is recommended prior to surgery

Staging objectives

- To determine extent of local tumour.
- To identify evidence of perineural spread.
- To identify evidence of skull base invasion.
- To identify lymph node metastases.

A combination of CT and MRI is often required for full imaging assessment. CT provides the detail regarding the bone margins of the sinus at risk, while MRI yields important information about the extent of soft tissue and perineural spread. The radiologist should be familiar with the pathways of spread and those critical areas of potential tumour spread that influence operability and the choice of surgical technique.

Staging

CT

- 2-3 mm axial sections using spiral technique following injection of intravenous contrast medium through the skull base and primary tumour.
- Using MDCT, slice thickness will depend on scanner capability. In general, sections are acquired at 1.25-2.5 mm and reformatted no greater than 5 mm for viewing.
- 5 mm axial sections through the whole neck to assess lymph nodes.
- Coronal reformatted images are useful for pre-surgical planning.

Values of $CTDI_{vol}$ should normally be below the relevant national reference dose for the region of scan and patient group (see Appendix and section on *Radiation Protection for the Patient in CT* in chapter 2).

44

MRI

MRI is best for assessing skull base invasion, soft-tissue intracranial extension and perineural spread.

Protocol for imaging of paranasal sinus tumours				
Sequence	Plane	Slice thickness	Field of view	Reason
STIR T1W T2W Fat Sat T1W	Coronal Coronal Axial Axial	3 mm (max) 3 mm 3 mm 5-6 mm	Small Small Small Small	Identification of primary tumour and survey of neck for nodes
T1W + Gad Fat Sat	Axial	5-6 mm	Small	To look for perineural spread
T1W + Gad Fat Sat	Coronal	3 mm	Small	Orbital extension (maxillary and ethmoid tumours) Intracranial & Cavernous sinus extension (sphenoid and ethmoid)
T1 + Gad Fat Sat	Sagittal	3 mm	Small	As required

Follow-up

Routine follow-up 3-4 months after completion of treatment is useful for establishing a baseline for future comparison. MRI is more helpful than CT, and evaluating radiologists should be familiar with the expected post-surgical changes.

Tip

- Differentiation of tumour from retained secretions can be difficult, and is best achieved with contrast-enhanced MRI.

Hypopharynx

Clinical background

The hypopharynx extends from the hyoid bone superiorly down to the postcricoid region inferiorly. It includes the posterior pharyngeal wall, the piriform sinuses and the postcricoid region. Over 95% of tumours arising here are of squamous cell type. Bulky submucosal spread is typical (resulting in clinical understaging at endoscopy) and the majority have lymph node metastases to the neck at presentation. Definitive treatment may involve surgery or radiotherapy.

Who should be imaged?

All patients with biopsy-proven hypopharynx cancer require MRI for staging.

45

Staging objectives

- To determine extent of local tumour.
- To identify evidence of midline involvement.
- To identify evidence of cartilage invasion.
- To identify lymph node metastases.
- To identify involvement of apex of piriform sinus

Staging

MRI

Contrast-enhanced MRI is the preferred technique because of its multiplanar imaging capabilities and superior soft tissue contrast.

Protocol for imaging of paranasal sinus tumours				
Sequence	Plane	Slice thickness	Field of view	Reason
STIR T1W T2W Fat Sat T1W	Coronal Coronal Axial Axial	3 mm (max) 3 mm 3 mm 5-6 mm	Small Small Small Small	Identification of primary tumour and survey of neck for nodes
T1W + Gad Fat Sat	Axial	5-6 mm	Small	
T1W + Gad Fat Sat	Coronal	3 mm	Small	

CT

- 2-3 mm axial sections using spiral technique from hard palate to supraclavicular fossa following intravenous contrast medium enhancement.
- Using MDCT, slice thickness will depend on scanner capability. In general, sections are acquired at 1.25-2.5 mm and reformatted no greater than 3-5 mm for viewing.

Values of $CTDI_{vol}$ should normally be below the relevant national reference dose for the region of scan and patient group (see Appendix and section on *Radiation Protection for the Patient in CT* in chapter 2).

PET-CT

[18]FDG PET-CT is useful for determining the extent of primary disease and also for re-staging post-treatment disease recurrence.

Follow-up

Follow-up imaging 2-3 months after treatment is useful to establish a baseline for future comparison.

Salivary glands

Clinical background

The major salivary glands are the 3-paired parotid, submandibular and sublingual glands. Generally, the smaller the salivary gland, the more likely it is that any tumour arising within it will be malignant. Thus, benign parotid tumours are not that uncommon and are often [18]FDG PET-positive. Tumours in the parotid glands arise from a variety of tissue elements, but superficial lobe tumours are more likely to be benign, while deep lobe tumours are often malignant. Malignant parotid tumours tend to be painful, rapidly growing and associated with facial nerve paralysis. The commonest benign parotid tumours are the pleomorphic adenoma (usually solitary) and Warthin's tumour (frequently multiple and bilateral). Mucoepidermoid and adenocystic carcinomas are the most common malignant tumours. Lymph node spread is less common than with other head and neck tumours, and distant spread is usually to the lungs. The parotid has a rich network of lymphatic vessels and intra-parotid nodal involvement is often the site of metastatic disease, particularly from scalp tumours. Parotid nodal enlargement may also be seen in lymphoma. Treatment of malignant disease is usually a combination of surgery and adjuvant radiotherapy.

Who should be imaged?

All patients with biopsy-proven or suspected salivary gland tumours require imaging with MRI.

Staging objectives

- To determine extent of local tumour.
- To identify lymph node metastases to the neck.

Staging

MRI

MRI is the imaging modality of choice for staging salivary gland tumours. The soft tissue resolution and multiplanar imaging are necessary for surgical planning and radiation field planning.

Protocol for imaging of salivary gland tumours				
Sequence	Plane	Slice thickness	Field of view	Reason
STIR T1W T2W Fat Sat T1W	Coronal Coronal Axial Axial	3 mm (max) 3 mm 3 mm 5-6 mm	Small Small Small Small	Identification of primary tumour and survey of neck for nodes
T1W + Gad Fat Sat	Axial	5-6 mm	Small	To look for perineural spread
T1W + Gad Fat Sat	Coronal	3 mm	Small	To look for perineural spread Assess intracranial extension

PET-CT

The salivary glands usually demonstrate moderate physiological [18]FDG uptake on PET-CT. Furthermore, salivary gland tumours can have a variable appearance on [18]FDG PET-CT and some tumours do not demonstrate any significant [18]FDG uptake. Therefore, the technique does not have a major role in the assessment of primary salivary tumours.

Follow-up

Follow-up MRI is useful 2-3 months after completion of treatment to establish a baseline for future comparison.

Tips

- Intraparotid lymph nodes can mimic primary salivary tumours on imaging.
- Tumour characterisation is usually not required for management.
- Intraparotid lymph node enlargement due to other malignancies such as lymphoma is clearly shown on [18]FDG PET-CT.

Oral cavity & oropharynx

Clinical background

Squamous cell tumours are the commonest histological subtype of tumours of the oral cavity and oropharynx and are associated with tobacco and alcohol exposure. Staging systems are based more on tumour size than on depth or extent, although it is the depth of invasion that determines the primary therapeutic approach.

In the oral cavity, most tumours tend to arise along the dependent portions. Most floor of mouth tumours occur within 2 cm of the midline. Tongue tumours usually arise from the lateral aspects of the posterior two-thirds of the tongue. Buccal mucosal tumours generally arise from the inner aspects of the cheeks. Gingival tumours arise from the mucous membrane covering the floor of mouth, mandible and maxilla, and have well-defined patterns of spread that define their surgical management. The retromolar trigone is a small triangular region posterior to the last molars and tumours arising here have complex patterns of spread. Tongue base tumours are often clinically silent and often present with neck lymphadenopathy.

The treatment of these tumours involves a combination of surgery and adjuvant radiotherapy. Neoadjuvant chemo-radiotherapy is under assessment.

Who should be imaged?

All patients with biopsy-proven or suspected malignant oral disease should be imaged using MRI.

Staging objectives

- To determine extent of local tumour.
- To identify evidence of deep invasion particularly of the masticator space, tongue and into the submandibular space.
- To identify evidence of bone invasion of the mandible and maxillary.
- To identify lymph node metastases to the neck.

Staging

MRI

MRI is the preferred imaging technique and is highly dependent on the site of the primary tumour. Sequences should involve those through the neck and the primary site.

Protocol for imaging of salivary gland tumours				
Sequence	Plane	Slice thickness	Field of view	Reason
STIR T1W T2W Fat Sat T1W	Coronal Coronal Axial Axial	3 mm (max) 3 mm 3 mm 5-6 mm	Small Small Small Small	Identification of primary tumour and survey of neck for nodes
T1W + Gad Fat Sat	Axial	5-6 mm	Small	
T1W + Gad Fat Sat	Coronal	3 mm	Small	
T1 + Gad	Sagittal	3 mm	Small	Tongue base tumours
Fat Sat				Epiglottic extension

PET-CT

The normal palatine tonsils are almost always identified on ^{18}FDG PET-CT, showing moderate uptake of ^{18}FDG. There is overlap between these physiological appearances and uptake observed in primary malignancy, but asymmetrical uptake (in the absence of a tonsillectomy) in the correct clinical context should raise suspicion (see also section in chapter 23 - carcinoma of unknown primary origin). ^{18}FDG PET-CT may be useful for nodal staging.

Follow-up

Follow-up MRI is useful 2-3 months after completion of treatment to establish a baseline for future comparison.

Tips

- Superficial mucosal tumours of the tongue and buccal mucosa can be difficult to visualise.

- The orthopantomogram is an important complementary imaging technique for assessment of bone involvement of the mandible.

- Intense uptake of ^{18}FDG can be observed in inflammatory conditions.

Thyroid cancer

Clinical background

Clinical thyroid cancer is uncommon (0.5% of all cancer deaths) although there is a high frequency of occult tumours identified at post-mortem. Most thyroid cancers are relatively indolent tumours that have a chronic clinical course with infrequent metastatic disease. Papillary cancer is the most common histological type and is more frequent in iodine-rich areas.

It is the main cancer induced by radiation exposure in childhood and characteristically has low-grade malignant potential. Lymph node spread is a feature but often remains localised to the nodes without further spread. Distant spread is uncommon and the prognosis is generally excellent. Follicular cancer tends to occur in iodine-deficient areas. Unlike papillary cancer, follicular cancer rarely spreads to the nodes but can metastasise to the lungs, bones and liver. Anaplastic cancer is the most aggressive type with a poor prognosis. Medullary cancer can be sporadic or familial, and the serum calcitonin levels are usually elevated.

Treatment depends on the histological type of tumour. Papillary cancers are treated surgically and radioiodine ablation can only be used post-operatively when all residual thyroid tissue has been removed. Follicular cancers are managed by total thyroidectomy and radio-ablation. Anaplastic cancers usually require radiotherapy. Medullary cancers are treated by surgery and / or radiotherapy in the early stages with chemotherapy for advanced disease.

Who should be imaged?

For low volume and early stage disease pre-operative imaging is seldom required as surgery is the primary management. MRI or CT scanning is indicated when there is suspicion of tumour extension into the larynx, trachea or retrosternally into the mediastinum. MRI is the preferred imaging technique because the iodine contrast used for CT scanning may delay post-operative radio-iodine therapy.

Staging objectives

- To determine extent of local tumour.
- To identify lymph node metastases to the neck.
- To identify evidence of metastatic spread.

Both CT and MRI are used for thyroid cancer staging but contrast-enhanced CT may not be appropriate if management is to include diagnostic and therapeutic scanning with Iodine[131].

Staging

MRI

MRI is the preferred imaging of choice for determining the local extent of thyroid cancer. Axial and coronal sequences with gadolinium enhancement are used as for other head and neck tumour sites. For patients who are claustrophobic and cannot tolerate MRI, CT imaging with gadolinium contrast enhancement should be performed.

Protocol for imaging of thyroid tumours				
Sequence	Plane	Slice thickness	Field of view	Reason
STIR T1W T2W Fat Sat T1W	Coronal Coronal Axial Axial	3 mm (max) 3 mm 3 mm 5-6 mm	Small Small Small Small	Identification of primary tumour and survey of neck for nodes
T1W + Gad Fat Sat	Axial	5-6 mm	Small	
T1W + Gad Fat Sat	Coronal	3 mm	Small	
T1W + Gad Fat Sat	Sagittal	3 mm	Small	Tongue base tumours Epiglottic extension

CT

The entire neck should be scanned to include the supraclavicular fossae using 5 mm thick sections. It should be clearly indicated by the referring clinician whether or not iodine contrast enhancement can be used. The thorax may be scanned without intravenous contrast to identify pulmonary metastases.

- Using MDCT, slice thickness will depend on scanner capability. In general, sections are acquired at 1.25-2.5 mm and reformatted no greater than 5 mm for viewing.

Values of $CTDI_{vol}$ should normally be below the relevant national reference dose for the region of scan and patient group (see Appendix and section on *Radiation Protection for the Patient in CT* in chapter 2).

PET-CT

[18]FDG uptake is not usually observed in the normal thyroid gland. [18]FDG uptake by well-differentiated thyroid cancer is low but increased [18]FDG uptake is seen in moderately and poorly-differentiated histological types, such as Tall cell and Hurthle cell types. Poorly differentiated tumours show loss of iodine uptake and the observation of low iodine / high [18]FDG uptake and vice versa is termed the "flip-flop" phenomenon. The predominant indication for the use of [18]FDG PET-CT in thyroid cancer is in patients who have negative Iodine[131] scans with elevated serum thyroglobulin levels because PET-CT permits the detection and localisaton of non-iodine avid metastases.

Follow-up

Follow-up MRI is useful 2-3 months after completion of treatment to establish a baseline for future comparison.

Tips

- Most imaging is performed in the post-surgical setting to detect recurrences in patients with rising serum thyroglobulin.
- Careful review of the retrotracheal and retrosternal regions is required.
- May need to avoid contrast-enhanced CT if radioiodine ablation is under consideration.
- Diffuse increased uptake by the thyroid gland is an appearance most frequently observed in inflammation (thyroiditis).
- If focal intense [18]FDG uptake is seen in the thyroid gland it may either represent uptake by a benign nodule, by an occult primary thyroid malignancy, or by an intrathyroid metastasis. When focal increased uptake is observed in the thyroid, an ultrasound with or without FNA is always indicated.

51

CHAPTER 7

Lung cancer

Clinical background

Lung cancer is one of the commonest malignancies and a leading cause of death with a well-known and potentially avoidable carcinogen (tobacco). The disease is often diagnosed late with a 5-year survival of 15%. About 80% of lung cancer is of non-small-cell histology with the rest being of small-cell type. Almost half of all non-small cell lung cancer patients have predominantly intrathoracic disease and are treated either by surgery alone or with combination therapy (predominantly radiotherapy) with or without surgery. By contrast, 80% of small-cell lung cancer patients have metastatic disease and are treated principally with chemotherapy.

Treatment depends on the extent of disease, the location of the primary tumour and the presence or absence of co-morbid conditions. The main purpose of staging is to define which patients are suitable for curative treatment by defining the intrathoracic and extrathoracic extent of the disease. Thus, it is important to define the extent of the primary tumour and also the extent (volume and location) of nodal involvement: ipsilateral hilar and small volume ipsilateral mediastinal nodes may not preclude surgery, whereas bulky mediastinal nodes whether ipsilateral or contralateral usually preclude curative surgery.

The TNM staging system is used primarily for non-small cell lung cancer but is rarely used for small cell neoplasm either in clinical practice or in clinical trials; instead the commoner approach is to classify tumours as either "limited" (limited to one hemithorax) or "extensive" (extends outside the hemithorax) stage. Patients with pleural disease from small-cell disease are considered to have extensive disease.

Who should be imaged?

All patients with a diagnosis of lung cancer should be staged. The exception may be in those patients with a performance status such that only palliative therapy is to be undertaken. Even this group of patients, however, may require CT imaging to guide palliative radiotherapy.

Staging objectives

- To assess resectability for non small-cell lung cancer.
- To identify the size and extent of the local tumour.
- To assess mediastinal invasion and relationship of the tumour to the carina.
- To assess hilar and mediastinal adenopathy.
- To identify chest wall or vertebral body invasion.
- To identify distant metastases in the liver, adrenal glands and upper abdominal lymph nodes.
- To identify supraclavicular fossa nodes.

Staging

CT of the abdomen and chest is the investigation of choice to stage the primary tumour and to detect metastatic disease. CT of the brain should be included in the initial staging, if curative therapy is being considered or if symptoms are present. Many centres routinely scan the brain in all small-cell lung cancer patients as 10% will have asymptomatic metastatic disease at the time of diagnosis. MRI is the investigation of choice if the CT is normal in the presence of neurological signs.

CT

- Post-contrast scans through the chest (to include supraclavicular fossa) and upper abdomen (to include the liver and adrenal glands).
- 100-150 ml of intravenous iodinated contrast medium injected at 3-4 ml/sec.
- Scan delay of 20 seconds for optimal visualisation of the pulmonary artery and great vessels.
- Scan delay of 60-70 seconds for optimal visualisation of the liver in the portal venous phase is recommended.
- Using MDCT slice thickness will depend on scanner capability. In general, sections are acquired at 1.25-2.5 mm and reformatted at 5 mm for viewing.

Note:
Pancoast (superior sulcus) tumours are best visualised by multiplanar reconstructions and 3-D rendered images. However, the extent of these tumours is best demonstrated by MRI.

Values of $CTDI_{vol}$ should normally be below the relevant national reference dose for the region of scan and patient group (see Appendix and section on *Radiation Protection for the Patient in CT* in chapter 2).

MRI

- T1W axial, coronal and sagittal images with section thickness of 5-7 mm with an appropriate field of view are recommended.
- MR angiography can be performed, if vascular invasion suspected. Contrast enhancement with spectral fat suppression can also be useful.

PET-CT

[18]FDG PET-CT is increasingly being used to assess nodal involvement and distant metastases prior to definitive surgery. A positive mediastinal PET-CT, in an otherwise operable patient, should be confirmed by biopsy as false positive uptake can occur with granulomatous disease. It should also be remembered that false negative examinations can occur with low-grade adenocarcinoma,

carcinoid and bronchoalveolar cell carcinoma. These latter two tumours can have a highly variable appearance on [18]FDG PET-CT ranging from low grade uptake through to moderate or intense uptake in individual patients depending on the primary tumour grade. Brain metastases may be difficult to see on [18]FDG PET-CT due to normal physiological uptake of [18]FDG as a result of metabolic activity.

Guidelines have recently been published by NICE which state that all potential surgical patients should have a [18]FDG PET scan prior to surgery, and all patients planned for radical radiotherapy should also have a PET scan to assess whether there are any distant metastases.

Follow-up

Repeat staging should be undertaken after downstaging with chemotherapy prior to surgery. Repeat staging is also required for patients who develop symptoms of SVC obstruction.

Tips

- Some surgeons require a more detailed classification of nodal station involvement and the American Joint Committee on Cancer classification is often used for this purpose.
- Satellite nodules defined as additional nodules in the same lobe as the primary tumour but distinct from the primary lesion are classified as T4 disease. Pleural foci separate from primary pleural invasion by tumour is classified as T4 disease. Nodules in a different lobe (ipsilateral or contralateral) are considered to represent metastatic disease (M1).
- Vocal cord palsy, superior vena caval invasion, obstruction of the oesophagus or trachea are considered to represent T4 disease, if caused by the primary tumour, but if due to nodal disease are considered to be N2.

Lung metastases

Screening for pulmonary metastases is undertaken when early detection will have a major impact on treatment, e.g., testicular tumours, soft tissue sarcomas or bone tumours. Routine inclusion of the chest in staging head and neck tumours is more controversial and should be performed on a patient-by-patient basis.

CT

CT is the investigation of choice.

- Using MDCT slice thickness will depend on scanner capability. In general, sections are acquired at 1.25-2.5 mm and reformatted at 5 mm for viewing.

Values of CTDI$_{vol}$ should normally be below the relevant national reference dose for the region of scan and patient group (see Appendix and section on *Radiation Protection for the Patient in CT* in chapter 2).

Pleural mesothelioma

Clinical background

Malignant mesotheliomas are relatively rare and represent about 2% of all malignant tumours. The risk factor is exposure to asbestos, and the incidence of malignant mesothelioma is expected to continue to increase in the UK over the next 25 years. Many tumours are diagnosed at an advanced stage with a consequent poor prognosis. If diagnosed earlier, then surgery and chemotherapy offer potential cure. The histological cell type is important. Biopsy of the pleural tumour and radiotherapy to the portal site should be given to prevent seeding down the track. Epithelioid tumours are associated with the best prognosis, and desmoplastic tumours with the worst.

These tumours are staged using the TNM classification. T1 to T3 tumours are potentially resectable. Regional nodes include internal mammary, intrathoracic, scalene and supraclavicular nodes.

Who should be imaged?

Many patients are imaged prior to diagnosis as part of the investigation of recurrent pleural effusions. All patients whose performance status is suitable should be staged as surgery is now an option.

Staging objectives

- To assess the T- and N- stage to identify potential surgical candidates.
- To identify T4 tumours including spread transgression of the diaphragm as this will render the patient unsuitable for resection at any time.

Staging

CT of the abdomen and chest is the investigation of choice to stage the primary tumour and to detect distant spread.

CT

- Post-contrast scans through the chest (to include supraclavicular fossa) and upper abdomen (to include the liver and adrenal glands).
- 100-150 ml of intravenous iodinated contrast medium injected at 3-4 ml/sec.
- Scan delay of 50 seconds for optimal visualisation of the pleural tumour and also allowing assessment of the mediastinal nodes.
- Using MDCT slice thickness will depend on scanner capability. In general, sections are acquired at 1.25-2.5 mm and reformatted at 5 mm for viewing.

Values of $CTDI_{vol}$ should normally be below the relevant national reference dose for the region of scan and patient group (see Appendix and section on *Radiation Protection for the Patient in CT* in chapter 2).

PET-CT

[18]FDG PET-CT will identify the extent of tumour but may be difficult to interpret after talc pleurodesis as this will cause increased uptake in the pleura.

Follow-up

Repeat staging to assess response to chemotherapy, if this is given to downstage patients prior to surgery.

Tip

- CT of the chest and abdomen should be obtained as a single acquisition to enable the sagittal and coronal reformats of the entire diaphragm to be obtained at optimal contrast enhancement. These are the most appropriate images to interrogate in order to deter mine if diaphragmatic transgression has occurred.

CHAPTER 8

56

Oesophagus and stomach cancers

Oesophageal cancer

Clinical background

The incidence of oesophageal cancer is increasing and represents the third most common gastrointestinal malignancy. The majority of patients with adenocarcinoma of the oesophagus receive combined modality treatment in the form of either combination chemotherapy followed by surgery, or chemoradiotherapy followed by surgery. For patients presenting with squamous carcinoma of the oesophagus, the preferred mode of treatment is combination chemoradiotherapy. Primary oesophageal adenocarcinoma most commonly presents in the lower third of the oesophagus, and much less commonly in the mid- and upper-oesophagus, and is strongly associated with a hiatus hernia and reflux disease. Mediastinal, subcarinal, peri-oesophageal and perigastric nodal disease constitutes regional lymphadenopathy. For all oesophageal tumours, nodal disease at or below the level of the coeliac axis constitutes metastatic disease. For tumours arising above the thoracic inlet, namely in the cervical oesophagus, local regional lymph nodes are considered to be present in the peri-oesophageal, supraclavicular, cervical, internal jugular and the scalene territories.

Who should be imaged?

All patients with oesophageal cancer diagnosed at endoscopy or suspected following an upper gastrointestinal barium examination using fluoroscopy. In general, patients with dysplasia and without invasive cancer do not require full CT staging.

Staging objectives

- To define tumour position and estimate the proximal and distal extent of the tumour and length of tumour.

- To identify local invasion, particularly with respect to the trachea, main bronchi, aorta, pericardium, pleura, diaphragmatic hiatus and crura.

- To identify lymph node enlargement, particularly peri-oesophageal, mediastinal and perigastric regions.

- To identify metastases in retroperitoneal lymph nodes, in the liver and peritoneal cavity.

- To determine the degree of oesophageal obstruction and to identify the presence of complications such as localised perforation or fistulation.

Staging

CT of the thorax and abdomen is the primary imaging investigation.

CT

- Oral administration of 1 litre of water or iodinated contrast medium (see Tips).

- 100-150 ml of intravenous iodinated contrast medium injected at 3-4 ml/sec.

- MDCT is commenced at 20-25 seconds (chest) and 70-80 seconds (abdomen) post-injection.

- Using MDCT, slice thickness will depend on scanner capability. In general, sections are acquired at 1.25-2.5 mm and reformatted at 5 mm for viewing.

Values of $CTDI_{vol}$ should normally be below the relevant national reference dose for the region of scan and patient group (see Appendix and section on *Radiation Protection for the Patient in CT* in chapter 2).

PET-CT

^{18}FDG PET-CT is increasingly being used for primary tumour staging as oesophageal carcinoma is intensely ^{18}FDG avid and the technique is helpful for delineating the craniocaudal extent of oesophageal disease and also for detecting involved regional and distant nodes, and metastases.

Follow-up

CT is the primary imaging modality for follow-up with the same protocol, dictated by the type of treatment (combination chemotherapy, chemoradiotherapy, surgery). Following surgery a CT at 3 months is recommended as a baseline for further assessment. Subsequent imaging will depend on disease status and patient symptoms.

Tips

- The patient may be scanned prone to rule out invasion of the aortic adventitia.

- 200 ml of water given orally immediately before the patient is scanned may help to maximise oesophageal distension and visualisation of the endoluminal component of the tumour.

- Laparoscopy is required in all sub-diaphragmatic tumours in order to detect small volume peritoneal disease that may not be seen by imaging.

Stomach cancer

Clinical background

In patients presenting with symptoms of gastric cancer, approximately one-third will have metastatic disease with an associated 2% relative survival rate. Patients presenting with early stage disease may be curable with surgery, with survival varying from 50% to 15%. Patients receive neoadjuvant chemotherapy in addition to surgery for this disease.

The objective of gastric resection is to achieve clear histological margins and total gastrectomy is not necessary for all patients with gastric adenocarcinoma The extent of nodal dissection is defined as a major factor in staging and can influence outcome by stage. Although there is no benefit in routinely performing extended lymph node dissection in gastric cancer, for patients with N2 disease (left gastric, common hepatic and coeliac and splenic artery nodes), a more extended dissection may be of benefit. The precise role of imaging in the pre-operative and surgical management of gastric cancers has yet to be defined, although the delineation of extent of tumor as well as local spread will influence the type of surgery performed. Imaging is also essential to rule out metastatic disease in patients considered suitable for surgery. Currently, nodal staging is not sufficiently accurate to enable selection between patients who will require limited versus extended surgical lymph node dissection.

Who should be imaged?

All patients with gastric carcinoma.

Staging objectives

- To identify metastatic disease in the liver and peritoneum including ovarian deposits.
- To determine the proportion of stomach involved by tumour to assist with decision making with regard to the extent surgery to be performed.
- To identify the presence or absence of peritoneal nodules and nodal enlargement (peri-gastric, coeliac axis nodes versus metastatic nodal disease in retroperitoneum).
- To document the degree of outflow obstruction in order to guide the clinical management of obstructive symptoms.

Staging

CT of the thorax, abdomen and pelvis is the primary imaging investigation.

CT

- Oral administration of 1 litre of water as a contrast agent, of which 400 ml is to be drunk immediately prior to going onto the scanner (see Tips).
- To ensure maximum gastric distension (an anti-peristaltic agent is, in general, not required).
- MDCT is commenced at 20-25 seconds (chest) and 70-80 seconds (abdomen and pelvis) post-injection.
- Using MDCT, slice thickness will depend on scanner capability. In general, sections are acquired at 1.25-2.5 mm and reformatted at 5 mm for viewing.

Values of CTDI$_{vol}$ should normally be below the relevant national reference dose for the region of scan and patient group (see Appendix and section on *Radiation Protection for the Patient in CT* in chapter 2).

PET-CT

Although [18]FDG PET-CT can be a useful modality for the assessment of gastric carcinomas, the value of the technique in this disease appears to be less than that observed with oesophageal carcinoma. This is because the stomach often shows low to moderate grade physiological [18]FDG uptake and small local involved nodes may not demonstrate significant [18]FDG uptake.

Follow-up

CT is the primary imaging modality for follow-up with the same protocol, dictated by the type of treatment (combination chemotherapy, chemoradiotherapy, surgery). Following surgery, a CT at 3 months is recommended as a baseline for further assessment. Subsequent imaging will depend on disease status and patient symptoms.

Tips

- The patient may be scanned prone to aid assessment of local invasion.
- 400 ml of water given orally immediately before the patient is scanned may help to maximise gastric distension and visualisation of the luminal component of the tumour.
- Laparoscopy is required in all sub-diaphragmatic tumours in order to detect small volume peritoneal disease that may not be seen by imaging.

CHAPTER 9

Liver cancer

Liver metastases

Clinical background

The liver is the second most frequent metastatic site and, as a consequence, liver metastases represent the commonest form of malignant liver disease in the UK. The prevalence of benign liver tumours is also high, and it is clearly important that benign liver lesions are distinguished from malignant disease. Liver metastases usually indicate that the malignant disease is no longer localised and treatment is usually with systemic chemotherapy. In patients in whom the primary lesion has been or can be eradicated and the liver is the only site of disease then surgical resection or an ablative therapy may be considered. Liver resection and ablation are most commonly performed for colorectal metastases and neuroendocrine tumours but may be appropriate in selected cases from other malignancies, particularly if there has been a long interval between treatment of the primary tumour and representation with liver metastases. Cardiovascular fitness, the segmental distribution of lesions and vascular involvement are major determinants for resection, with lesion size and number influencing selection for ablation. Metastases within both lobes of the liver are not absolute contraindications to either resection or ablation.

Who should be imaged?

Neoplasms with a propensity to metastasise to the liver as indicated in the appropriate sections of these guidelines with the aim of detecting metastases. Focal liver lesions in this context also require individual characterisation when their nature will affect the nature of the treatment given.

Malignant disease confined to the liver in patients deemed fit for resection or ablative therapy should be imaged with a view to detect the number and location of individual lesions to aid in the planning of physical therapies.

Staging objectives

- To determine the presence of liver metastases in patients with a known primary malignancy (see appropriate sections).

- To identify the primary tumour if the liver lesion(s) have the imaging characteristics of metastases.

- To identify the distribution (number and location) of malignant lesions and their relationships to the major vascular structures.

- To identify other sites of metastatic disease in patients being considered for resection or ablative therapies.

- To evaluate whether the liver pathology is benign, primary malignant liver disease or metastatic and thereby to decide whether no treatment, radical surgery or chemotherapy is required.

- To avoid biopsy if the lesion(s) are potentially resectable and the patient is a candidate for liver resection.

- To identify the need for percutaneous-targeted biopsy which is generally required for systemic chemotherapy in the absence of a known primary or appropriate temporal relationship to a prior primary.

Staging

The liver is usually examined as part of the general staging of patients with malignant disease when appropriate clinical areas are imaged (see guidelines appropriate to the primary tumour). In general CT is used for this purpose. Liver-only MRI can also be used to identify all liver malignant lesions present in patients who are candidates for resection. [18]FDG PET-CT is likely to be of value in patients with colorectal cancer being considered for resection particularly as it can identify patients with extra-hepatic disease which may preclude hepatic surgery.

In general, liver-only examinations are performed. Contrast-enhanced ultrasound, multiphasic MDCT, and MRI can all be used to characterise focal liver lesions identified as incidental or indeterminate as part of initial staging. However, in most instances liver MRI with contrast medium usage will usually be the imaging modality of choice.

CT

- Oral administration of 1 litre of water or iodinated contrast medium.

- 100-150 ml of intravenous iodinated contrast medium injected at 3-4 ml/sec.

- MDCT through the liver is commenced at 65-70 seconds post-injection.

- Using MDCT, slice thickness will depend on scanner capability. In general, sections are acquired at 1.25-2.5 mm and reformatted at 5 mm for viewing.

- Additional late arterial phase (approximately 30-35 seconds post-injection) may be used for neuroendocrine tumours and hepatocellular carcinomas which are typically hypervascular (as are the benign lesions such as focal nodular hyperplasia and hepatocellular adenoma).

Some populations of liver metastases from renal cell carcinomas, melanomas, sarcomas and breast cancers are also hypervascular; however, the frequency of liver metastases, only visible on the arterial phase that will change the overall stage and affect management, is extremely low; thus additional arterial phase imaging in these patient groups is not routinely recommended.

61

MRI

- As breathing artefacts are problematic for liver imaging, strategies to overcome this need to be used in all patients. The appropriate strategy will depend on MRI machine specification but could include: breath-holding, navigator assisted, respiratory ordered phase encoding, and respiratory compensation.

- A multichannel surface coil should be used in all cases. The field of view will in general be the whole liver.

- It is to be noted that there is little general consensus with regard to optimal liver protocols mostly due to compromises that need to be made because of the MRI scanner being used.

- Most imagers would agree that the basic sequences that should be undertaken include T1W and T2W sequences. T1W sequences should be performed using spin- or gradient-echo sequences with the spins "in-phase" (such that liver-spleen contrast is maximised). Opposed-phase GRE sequences are also valuable for the assessment of the fatty liver. T2W sequences with moderate and heavy weighting are useful for lesion characterisation and should be undertaken where possible.

- Extracellular small molecular weight contrast medium given intravenously is of value in lesion characterisation and detection (see injection protocol below).

- There is an increasing number of liver-specific contrast agents and these have both characterisation and detection roles. Some studies have demonstrated that liver-specific contrast media have advantages over non-specific small molecular weight chelates in specific circumstances, including prior to liver resection. Liver-specific contrast agents require protocol modification. Agents that increase T1-relaxivity require the use of GRE T1W sequences (with/without fat suppression). Those that increase T2* relaxivity (superparamagnetic iron oxides - SPIO particles) require appropriately weighted T2*/ proton density weighted GRE sequences.

Suggested basic sequences and those for use with extracellular small molecular weight contrast medium given intravenously are given below. Sequences and timings related to liver specific contrast agent vary widely and radiologists using these agents should familiarise themselves on their appropriate usage.

Protocol for imaging of liver metastases			
Sequence	Plane	Slice thickness	Principle observations
Fast GRE / FSE	Axial / coronal / sagittal	10 mm	Overview and planning sequence
GRE T1W (in-and opposed-phase)	Axial	6 mm	Demonstrate and eliminate the effects of intrahepatic fat & to characterise lesions
T2W – (fast) spin-echo with moderate and long TE. Alternatives include STIR and HASTE sequences	Axial	6 mm	Identify and characterise cysts and haemangiomas
Dynamic contrast study T1 GRE Fat Sat *	Axial (± oblique coronal for vascular relationships)	2.5 ± 1 mm	To characterise and identify tumours to demonstrate vascular relationships

Unenhanced, arterial, portal venous phases. Equilibrium phase obtained with a 10 minute delay may be of value in characterising haemangiomas and cholangiocarcinomas

PET-CT

[18]FDG PET-CT is a useful complementary technique to MRI for hepatic lesion detection (see also comments above). Metastases of the order of 5 mm in diameter can be detected in such tumours as colorectal cancer but it should be remembered that normal liver uptake of [18]FDG can be heterogeneous. [18]FDG PET-CT is a valuable technique in the post-radiofrequency ablation setting, being an early indicator of complete / incomplete tumour destruction and an effective modality for follow-up. CT and MRI are less sensitive than [18]FDG PET-CT in this situation.

Follow-up

Follow-up is conducted:

- To assess response to chemotherapy and is therefore performed at a frequency to correspond with the chemotherapy regimes.

- When there is clinical or serum marker evidence of recurrence.

- After surgery or ablative therapy to identify small volume recurrent disease within the liver or lungs which may be amenable to further resection / ablation.

Tips

- The arterial phase is relatively short and optimal timing is affected by cardiac output. To optimise dynamic contrast-enhanced CT or MRI in which an arterial phase is required, either a test bolus or a delay triggered from aortic enhancement thresholds can be used.

- To increase lesion-liver contrast in CT, particularly in the arterial phase, relatively high flow rates and volumes of contrast are helpful (e.g., 150 ml at 5 ml/sec).

- In patients with fatty livers the sensitivity of CT to hypovascular lesions is reduced; depending on the clinical issues to be addressed, MRI should be considered. (Remember the axiom: "Fat is your foe on CT, but your friend on MRI"!).

Primary liver cancer

Clinical background

Hepatocellular carcinoma (HCC) is the commonest of the primary liver neoplasms. Although it is the fifth most common malignancy worldwide, it represents only 1% of primary malignancies in the UK. The incidence of both HCC and cholangiocarcinoma (the second most frequent primary liver neoplasm) is rising within the UK. HCC often occurs on the background of liver cirrhosis which adds to the difficulty in obtaining an accurate diagnosis and in local staging. Sporadic HCCs, arising in the absence of liver cirrhosis, tend to be large at presentation with a dominant tumour mass, with or without satellite nodules, and occur in an older population. Fibrolamellar HCC is a distinct primary liver tumour occurring in young adults without liver cirrhosis and with normal serum alpha-foetoprotein levels.

Screening of high-risk patients with cirrhosis using ultrasound and serum alpha-foetoprotein measurements is now undertaken in the UK. Differentiating HCC from dysplastic nodules, the precursors of HCC, can be difficult using only non-invasive techniques. In the absence of chronic liver disease or with cirrhosis and good functional reserve, resection is the treatment of choice. In the presence of cirrhosis and poor functional reserve, liver transplantation can be offered depending upon lesion size, number, and the absence of major vascular invasion. Other therapies include percutaneous ablative therapies and trans-arterial chemoembolisation. There is no effective systemic chemotherapy for HCC.

Who should be imaged?

Cirrhotic patients at high-risk of developing HCC in whom ultrasound and / or serum alpha-foetoprotein measurements indicate the possibility of an underlying malignant cause; the intension being to detect and characterise liver lesions. All patients with focal liver lesions, and who are potential candidates for curative treatment, require all lesions to be characterised and mapped. In the absence of an extra-hepatic primary tumour or with features of a primary hepatic neoplasm, malignant liver lesions require full staging

Staging objectives

- To identify the presence and location of the primary tumour and to detect multifocal liver involvement.
- To note the presence of vascular invasion.
- To identify lymph node enlargement.
- To determine the full extent of disease including deposits in the lungs, bones and peritoneum.
- To note whether parenchymal liver disease and portal hypertension are also present.
- To identify features of chronic liver disease.
- To evaluate whether the liver pathology is benign, pre-malignant or primary malignant and consequently to decide whether radical surgery, ablative therapy or palliation is required.
- To avoid biopsy if the lesion(s) are potentially resectable or if alpha-foetoprotein significantly elevated.

Staging

CT

CT of the chest, abdomen and pelvis is the investigation of choice.

- Oral administration of 1 litre of water or iodinated contrast medium.
- 100-150 ml of intravenous iodinated contrast medium injected at 3-4 ml/sec.
- MDCT with acquisition through the chest with dual phase acquisition of the liver commenced at 30-35 and 65-70 seconds post-injection the last acquisition continued through the pelvis.
- Using MDCT, slice thickness will depend on scanner capability. In general, sections are acquired at 1.25-2.5 mm and reformatted at 5 mm for viewing.
- If arterial anatomy is required prior to resection, an additional early arterial acquisition at 18-20 seconds with 1 mm collimation can be acquired although this is not routinely advocated.

Values of CTDI$_{vol}$ should normally be below the relevant national reference dose for the region of scan and patient group (see Appendix and section on *Radiation Protection for the Patient in CT* in chapter 2).

MRI

MRI has advantages over CT particularly for the evaluation of focal liver lesions in the cirrhotic liver.

Protocol for imaging of primary liver tumours			
Sequence	Plane	Slice thickness	Principle observations
Fast GRE / FSE	Axial / coronal / sagittal	10 mm	Overview and planning sequence
GRE T1W (in- and opposed-phase)	Axial	6 mm	Demonstrate and eliminate the effects of intrahepatic fat & to characterise lesions
T2W – (fast) spin-echo with moderate and long TE. Alternatives include STIR and HASTE sequences	Axial	6 mm	Identify and characterise cysts and haemangiomas
Dynamic contrast study T1 GRE Fat Sat *	Axial (± oblique coronal for vascular relationships)	2.5 ± 1 mm	To characterise and identify tumours to demonstrate vascular relationships

* Unenhanced, arterial, portal venous phases. Equilibrium phase obtained with a 10 minute delay may be of value in characterising haemangiomas and cholangiocarcinomas

In patients with liver cirrhosis, contrast agents can be used either singly (usually extracellular small molecular weight contrast medium given intravenously) or in combination (usually SPIO particles) to exploit differences that exist in vascularity, hepatocytes function, or Kuppfer's cell density in order to differentiate between regenerative, dysplastic and neoplastic nodules.

PET-CT

[18]FDG PET-CT has variable efficacy in hepatobiliary tumours. The sensitivity for detection of hepatomas is in the range of 50-70%. Variable uptake of [18]FDG is seen in cholangiocarcinoma although certain histological subtypes such as nodular cholangiocarcinoma can demonstrate sensitivity in the region of 85%. False positive [18]FDG uptake is seen in acute cholangitis and inflammatory uptake is also observed following biliary stent insertion. Therefore when [18]FDG PET-CT is used for the assessment of cholangiocarcinoma it is generally important to perform the PET-CT study prior to biliary stent insertion.

Follow-up

Imaging follow-up is conducted:

- After surgery or ablative therapy to identify small volume recurrent disease which may be amenable to further resection / ablation.
- To assess response to chemo-embolisation.
- To assess the significance of indeterminate hypervascular lesions.

Tips

- With dynamic extracellular small molecular weight contrast medium enhancement it is important to have an unenhanced acquisition of the same sequence to identify true arterial enhancement; in liver cirrhosis, dysplastic nodules are often of high signal intensity.

- Sub-centimetre hypervascular lesions only identified on the arterial phase in patients with cirrhosis should be interpreted with caution – not all hypervascular lesions will be small HCCs.

- While the majority of HCCs are hypervascular, a minority are hypovascular.

- Well-differentiated HCCs may take up liver-specific contrast agents, while poorly-differentiated tumours usually do not; evaluation of all sequences with appropriate clinical parameters, including serum alpha-foetoprotein levels, is important in characterising focal liver lesions.

- Enlargement of lymph nodes is common in the presence of cirrhosis and, therefore, caution should be used in interpreting such peri-portal nodes as being involved.

66

CHAPTER 10

Pancreas

Clinical background

Pancreatic cancer constitutes 3% of all cancers in the UK. The commonest histological type is ductal adenocarcinoma which has a predilection for the pancreatic head and neck. Patients often present with obstructive jaundice. Ampullary carcinomas and distal common bile duct carcinomas may be indistinguishable from pancreatic head ductal adenocarcinomas but, despite having separate pathological staging systems, the therapeutic issues and work-up are identical.

Primary treatment is surgical in which all macroscopic tumour can be excised. CT and MRI are similar in their capability to assess local tumour extent with both tending to underestimate disease extent. Resection can be considered in the absence of metastatic disease or involvement of the visceral arteries or the portal venous structures. In selected cases short segments of the superior mesenteric or portal vein may be resected. Liver metastases, which are often small, and peritoneal metastases preclude resection. CT and MRI are poor predictors of lymph node involvement. Ideally, staging and resection are performed without prior stenting of bile ducts. The prognosis following resection is poor with 5-year survival less than 10%.

Percutaneous biopsy should not be performed in potentially resectable cases but usually performed prior to chemotherapy. Biliary drainage is usually the major palliative procedure required. Chemotherapy and radiotherapy have limited and predominantly palliative roles. Endoscopic ultrasound (EUS) is of value in problem-solving with small tumours, may allow biopsy without breaching the peritoneum and enable coeliac axis neural blocks to be done for pain relief.

Neuroendocrine tumours and cystic neoplasms of the pancreas are less common but have a more favourable prognosis. Neuroendocrine pancreatic tumours may present as a consequence of a hyper-functioning syndrome (often small tumours), as a non-functioning mass, or as part of Multiple Endocrine Neoplasia type 1 (may be multiple tumours).

Who should be imaged?

If a pancreatic neoplasm is suspected, either clinically or as a consequence of a prior investigation, diagnostic CT should be performed using a staging protocol. Pancreatic neoplasms may present with non-specific symptoms and therefore may be detected on CT undertaken as a survey abdominal scan. Such tumours are often advanced and recall for a dedicated staging CT is often unnecessary.

Staging objectives

- To determine evidence of involvement of the visceral arteries and portal venous system.
- To identify deposits in the liver and peritoneum.
- To detect lymph node enlargement.
- To identify bile duct and duodenal obstruction.
- To evaluate whether the pancreatic pathology is inflammatory or malignant and thereby
- To decide pre-operatively whether radical surgery is required.

Staging

Ultrasound is the primary investigation in identifying biliary obstruction as the cause of jaundice. CT is the investigation of choice if a pancreatic neoplasm is suspected. MRI is an alternative if a tumour is identified at MRCP, or to problem-solve if there are indeterminate features relating to the pancreas or liver on CT. EUS is also of value in problem-solving, particularly with small focal pancreatic lesions.

CT

- Oral administration of 1 litre of water as a contrast agent to fill the stomach and duodenum.
- 100-150 ml of intravenous iodinated contrast medium injected at 3-4 ml/sec.
- MDCT (dual phase acquisition) commenced at 35-40 seconds (pancreatic phase) and 65-70 seconds (portal venous phase) after onset of injection.
- Using MDCT images should be acquired at 1-1.25 mm slice thickness in the pancreatic phase and 2 mm in the portal venous phase.

Values of $CTDI_{vol}$ should normally be below the relevant national reference dose for the region of scan and patient group (see Appendix and section on *Radiation Protection for the Patient in CT* in chapter 2).

MRI

A negative oral contrast agent is helpful with a phased array surface coil.

Protocol for imaging of pancreatic tumours				
Sequence	Plane	Slice thickness	Field of view	Principle observations
Fast T2W imaging	Axial	10 mm	Liver and Pancreas	Overview and sequence planning
GRE T1W (in- and opposed-phase)	Axial	6 mm		Demonstrate and eliminate the effects of intrahepatic fat & characterise lesions

		6 mm liver		Identify characterise
T2W Short and Long TE or HASTE	Axial	4 mm pancreas		liver lesions Identify neuroendocrine pancreatic tumours
MRCP SSFSE	Coronal	5 cm		Demonstrate ductal anatomy If necessary supplement with 3-D FSE or 2-4 mm HASTE
T1W with fat saturation	Axial	5 mm	Pancreas	To identify small primary tumours
Dynamic contrast medium enhanced study 2-D / 3-D T1 GRE with or without fat saturation	Axial / oblique coronal * *see Tips	2.5 ± 1 mm	Liver and Pancreas	To delineate the primary tumour, vascular involvement and identify liver metastases

PET-CT

On [18]FDG PET-CT scans, acute pancreatitis and pancreatic carcinoma both show increased [18]FDG uptake, and it is therefore not possible to differentiate these conditions, although there may be some value to PET imaging when distinguishing chronic pancreatitis from carcinoma. [18]FDG PET-CT is not indicated routinely in pancreatic cancer but has been used to a limited extent to exclude distant metastases in patients being considered for radical treatment.

Follow-up

Routine imaging after surgery is not warranted as palliative chemotherapy is generally only considered when there is symptomatic disease. Follow-up imaging is conducted when there is clinical evidence of recurrence. Follow-up is performed to assess response to chemotherapy (+/- radiotherapy) and is, therefore, performed at a frequency to correspond with the chemotherapy regimes.

Tips

- Coronal or sagittal reformatted CT images can be very useful to evaluate vascular involvement. More complex reconstructions such as curved planar reformats are occasionally helpful.

- With the dynamic gadolinium-enhanced MR series, the optimal plane depends upon the location of the tumour. The pancreatic and portal venous phase acquisitions are best acquired using an oblique coronal plane for pancreatic head tumours followed by an axial acquisition. For tumours of the body and tail and for neuroendocrine tumours the initial acquisitions are best obtained axially. This is less critical if 3-D techniques are employed, because an isotropic dataset can be obtained that can be reconstructed in any plane.

- A delayed axial acquisition through the pancreas at 10 minutes is of value in neuroendocrine tumours.

- 3-D T1 with fat saturation is preferable to 2-D sequences for MRCP, because image quality is much improved.

CHAPTER 11

Colon, rectum and anal canal cancer

Colon cancer

Clinical background

Colorectal cancer is the second commonest cause of cancer death in the Western world. Pre-operative management of colonic cancer comprises pre-operative investigation including only colonoscopy and abdominal ultrasound or computed tomography before primary surgery and consideration for adjuvant therapy post-operatively. For the vast majority of patients, primary surgical resection will be the treatment of choice. Although there is currently no universally accepted pre-operative strategy for patients with colon cancer, it is known that T4 stage, N2 stage (4 or more malignant nodes), extramural venous invasion, and emergency clinical presentations are independent predictors of poor patient prognosis.

The lymphatic vessels run close to the vessels in the mesocolon and beneath the peritoneum of the posterior abdominal wall. There are three main groups of lymph nodes. The first group is the paracolic lymph nodes which lie in the peritoneum close to the colon. The second group lies along the main vessels supplying blood to the colon. The third group is the para-aortic nodes which cluster around the root of the superior mesenteric artery and inferior mesenteric artery; retroperitoneal lymphadenopathy constitutes metastatic disease in colon cancer. Radiologists should be aware that the patterns of lymphatic spread are highly dependent on the primary tumour site so, for example, right colon cancers have lymphatic spread along the small bowel mesentery, and rectosigmoid tumours spread initially along the inferior mesenteric vessels.

Who should be imaged?

All patients with colon cancer diagnosed at endoscopy or suspected following a lower gastrointestinal barium examination using fluoroscopy.

Staging objectives

- To identify potential surgically difficult cases, e.g., tumours that infiltrate into adjacent structures and those presenting with bowel perforation.

- To determine the size and local extent of tumour and to note the degree of pericolic infiltration.

- To identify extension of tumour into adjacent structures such as abdominal wall, peritoneum, solid organs.

- To identify complications, such as the presence of bowel obstruction or perforation.

- To note the presence and extent of local pericolic nodal enlargement and to detect more distant nodal metastases. Nodes in the retro-peritoneum, pelvis and inguinal regions are considered to be metastatic.

- To identify the extent of metastatic disease in distant organs including the lungs and liver.

Staging

CT of the thorax, abdomen and pelvis is the primary imaging investigation. Abdominal ultrasound alone is not regarded as sufficient.

CT

- Oral administration of 1 litre of water or iodinated contrast medium to delineate small and large bowel.

- 100-150 ml of intravenous iodinated contrast medium injected at 3-4 ml/sec.

- MDCT is commenced at 20-25 seconds (chest) and 70-80 seconds (abdomen and pelvis) post-injection.

- Using MDCT, slice thickness will depend on scanner capability. In general, sections are acquired at 1.25-2.5 mm and reformatted at 5 mm for viewing.

Values of $CTDI_{vol}$ should normally be below the relevant national reference dose for the region of scan and patient group (see Appendix and section on *Radiation Protection for the Patient in CT* in chapter 2).

PET-CT

[18]FDG PET-CT is an accurate modality for detecting local recurrence as well as hepatic and extrahepatic recurrence. The technique has a major role in patients with hepatic recurrence who are being considered for surgical resection in order to exclude extrahepatic sites of disease (e.g., nodal and peritoneal). [18]FDG PET-CT is also an accurate modality for defining the presence of recurrent disease in the context of unexplained rising tumour markers.

Follow-up

Follow-up is undertaken when there is the suspicion of recurrent disease, e.g., elevation of serum carcinoembryonic antigen (CEA) levels, which should also be performed as a baseline prior to chemotherapy.

Tip

- A proportion of patients will present with metastatic disease to lungs or liver and, in these patients, careful assessment of metastatic disease will help to plan for subsequent metastectomy.

Rectal cancer

Clinical background

Rectal cancers have traditionally been thought to fare worse than colonic cancers, due to higher local recurrence rates, and have had poorer overall survival rates. However, with the introduction of better surgical techniques (total mesorectal excision), superior pre-operative imaging (high resolution MRI) and neoadjuvant treatments (radiotherapy and chemoradiotherapy), rectal cancer local recurrence rates have reduced and overall 5-year survival rates have increased to match the traditionally more favourable colonic cancer outcomes. As with colon cancers, patients presenting with obstruction or perforation have a worse prognosis. In addition, there are several poor prognostic features that are unique to the rectal site that can be identified pre-operatively by imaging. These include increasing depth of extramural tumour spread, involvement of the potential surgical resection margin, N2 nodal disease, extramural venous invasion, and T4 peritoneal perforation. For the vast majority of tumours, nodal spread is along the superior and middle rectal vessels and nodal metastases are confined to within the mesorectum. In a small percentage of cases (less than 10%) nodal metastases occur outside the mesorectum via the internal iliac chain with lateral spread to the pelvic sidewall or retroperitoneal lymphadenopathy. The pre-operative treatment strategy is tailored to the detailed local staging features of the primary tumour, taking into account the presence or absence of poor prognostic features, including the likelihood of achieving total mesorectal excision with clear circumferential resection margins.

Who should be imaged?

All patients with rectal-adenocarcinoma for whom total mesorectal excision surgery may be offered. Depending on the pre-operative treatment policy of the Colorectal MDT, upper rectal and sigmoid tumours may be staged using MRI

Staging objectives

- To identify potentially irresectable disease, namely tumour at or beyond the mesorectal fascia.

- To determine the length of tumour and location with respect to height above the anal verge.

- To determine the degree of local spread within the mesorectum and the presence of adverse features such as nodal spread, extramural venous invasion and peritoneal infiltration.

- To identify the presence of complications such as obstruction or perforation.

- To identify nodes outside the mesorectum which are considered metastatic, if in the external and common iliac regions. Internal iliac nodes are considered regional.

- To assess lungs and liver for presence of metastatic disease and to determine whether metastases are potentially resectable.

Staging

CT

CT of the thorax, abdomen and pelvis with intravenous contrast medium should be performed to detect distant spread of disease.

- Oral administration of 1 litre of water or iodinated contrast medium to delineate small and large bowel.

- 100-150 ml of intravenous iodinated contrast medium injected at 3-4 ml/sec.

- MDCT is commenced at 20-25 seconds (chest) and 70-80 seconds (abdomen and pelvis) post-injection.

- Using MDCT, slice thickness will depend on scanner capability. In general, sections are acquired at 1.25-2.5 mm and reformatted at 5 mm for viewing.

Values of $CTDI_{vol}$ should normally be below the relevant national reference dose for the region of scan and patient group (see Appendix and section on *Radiation Protection for the Patient in CT* in chapter 2).

MRI

MRI of the pelvis at 1.5 Tesla ; an abdomino-pelvic surface coil should be used. Anti-peristaltics may be helpful in a minority of cases (e.g. female patients post-hysterectomy).

Protocol for imaging of rectal cancer				
Sequence	Plane	Slice thickness	Field of view	Principle observations
T2W	Sagittal	5 mm	Large	Localise tumour Height of tumour above anal verge Length of tumour
T2W	Axial	5 mm	Large	Pelvic disease outside mesorectum
T2W	Oblique axial / coronal	3 mm	Small 16 cm fov	Tumour spread within mesorectum

PET-CT

[18]FDG PET-CT is an accurate modality for detecting local recurrence as well as hepatic and extrahepatic recurrence. The technique has a major role in patients with hepatic recurrence who are being considered for surgical resection in order to exclude extrahepatic sites of disease (e.g., nodal and peritoneal). [18]FDG PET-CT is also an accurate modality for defining the presence of recurrent disease in the context of unexplained rising tumour markers.

Follow-up

Follow-up is undertaken when there is the suspicion of recurrent disease, e.g., elevation of serum carcinoembryonic antigen (CEA) levels, which should also be performed as a baseline prior to chemotherapy.

Tips

When reporting MRI scans the following key findings should be mentioned:

- Site of Tumour – upper / mid / lower third.

- Height from anal verge and craniocaudal.

- Relationship to important landmarks, e.g., peritoneal reflection / seminal vesicles.

- Infiltrating border – smooth or nodular infiltration.
- Presence or absence of extramural venous invasion.
- Maximum depth of extramural spread.
- Presence or absence of malignant lymph nodes.
- Minimum distance to mesorectal fascia.
- In the final assessment, the TNM stage and an assessment of potential resection margin involvement (classified as at risk or safe) should be made.

Anal canal cancer

Clinical background

Carcinoma of the anal canal is a relatively uncommon cancer, accounting for less than 2% of large bowel malignancies and 1-6% of all anorectal tumours. Its incidence has been reported to be approximately 0.5 per 100,000 in males and 1.0 per 100,000 in females. There has been a slight increase in the incidence of the disease over the past few years in Denmark, Sweden and the United States of America.

Cancer arising from the anal canal can originate anywhere between the anorectal junction above and the anal verge below. The anal verge represents the junction between modified squamous epithelium of the anal canal and the anal skin. The majority of cancers arising from the anal canal are squamous cell carcinoma. Treatment with a combination of chemotherapy and radiotherapy is curative in the majority of patients with squamous cell carcinoma of the anus, without the need for radical surgery. However, radical surgery, such as abdomino-perineal resection, may still be necessary to treat local failure or recurrence following chemoradiation. Lymph node spread is generally along the external iliac channels to the inguinal lymph nodes, although for extensive primary disease internal iliac nodal disease and mesorectal nodal spread are well documented.

Who should be imaged?

All patients with biopsy-proven anal cancer. Patients with AIN (anal neoplasia in situ) probably do not require staging.

Staging objectives

- To assess local extent of disease prior to chemoradiation, to assist with radiotherapy planning, and to provide a baseline for follow-up.
- To determine presence or absence of locoregional lymphadenopathy.
- To assess for distant metastases.

Staging

CT

CT of the abdomen and pelvis (to cover groin areas) with intravenous contrast medium should be performed to detect distant spread of disease.

- Oral administration of 1 litre of water or iodinated contrast medium to delineate small and large bowel.

- 100-150 ml of intravenous iodinated contrast medium injected at 3-4 ml/sec.

- MDCT is commenced at 20-25 seconds (chest) and 70-80 seconds (abdomen and pelvis) post-injection.

- Using MDCT, slice thickness will depend on scanner capability. In general, sections are acquired at 1.25-2.5 mm and reformatted at 5 mm for viewing.

Values of $CTDI_{vol}$ should normally be below the relevant national reference dose for the region of scan and patient group (see Appendix and section on *Radiation Protection for the Patient in CT* in chapter 2).

MRI
MRI of the pelvis at 1.5 Tesla; an abdomino-pelvic surface coil should be used.

Protocol for imaging of anal canal cancer				
Sequence	Plane	Slice thickness	Field of view	Principle observations
T2W	Sagittal	5 mm	Large	Localise tumour Height of tumour above anal verge Length of tumour
T2W	Axial	5 mm	Large	Pelvic disease
T2W	Oblique axial and coronal series	3 mm	Small 16 cm fov	Tumour spread in relation to sphincter complex

Follow-up

Follow-up should be undertaken if relapse is suspected on clinical grounds.

Tips

- STIR sequences may be useful in delineating the tumour, but with improved T2W imaging techniques the tumour is frequently well delineated with this sequence alone.

- The T2W technique also has the advantage of showing fibrosis as low signal intensity which enables assessment of post-treatment related changes on subsequent follow-up imaging.

CHAPTER 12

Renal and adrenal tumours

Renal cell carcinoma

Clinical background

Renal cell carcinoma occurs in 11 out of 100,000 individuals with a true increase in its incidence in recent decades. It accounts for 80-90% of primary malignancies of the kidney in adults, the majority of which contain clear cells that are lipid and glycogen-rich. A less common variant is papillary cystadenocarcinoma (10-15%) and this has a less aggressive course. Accurate assessment of venous invasion is essential for planning surgery as, if present, the upper extent of tumour thrombus within the IVC (inferior vena cava) is vital information. Metastases are a strong indicator of a poor prognosis, and common sites include the lungs, bones and adrenal glands. Detection of all metastatic sites pre-operatively is important because the role of nephrectomy in such patients is limited. The para-aortic and paracaval nodes are the regional lymph nodes, and spread to these or beyond the peri-renal fascia markedly reduces patients' survival. [Note: Over recent years, nephron-sparing surgery has been increasingly used for tumours less than 4 cm as they have a less than 5% risk of being multicentric, and show a lower recurrence rate and improved survival after nephron-sparing surgery compared to larger tumours.]

Who should be imaged?

All patients in whom renal cell carcinoma is suspected on other imaging techniques should be imaged using CT. MRI is usually reserved for particular questions regarding venous invasion.

Staging objectives

- To identify the presence and extent of venous invasion including the ipsilateral renal vein and inferior vena cava. Where caval extension is present, it is important to determine the upper level of the extent of the thrombus in relation to the hepatic veins.

- To assess the size of the tumour.

- To assess perinephric tumour invasion.

- To identify local and regional lymph node involvement.

- To detect spread into adjacent structures including the liver, spleen and muscles.

- To identify involvement of the ipsilateral and contralateral adrenal glands.

- To identify tumours in the contralateral kidney.

In small tumours, additional objectives include assessing the feasibility of nephron-sparing surgery and therefore includes:

- An evaluation of the relationship of the tumour to the collecting system of the kidney and the kidney's arterial and venous supply.

- Providing optimal images to aid local surgical removal, e.g., volume-rendered 3-D for laparoscopic removal of small tumours.

Staging

CT

CT of the abdomen and chest is the investigation of choice to stage the primary tumour and to detect metastatic disease; the pelvis only needs to be included if there are symptoms referable to this, e.g., bone pain.

- Pre-contrast scans through the abdomen, in order to study contrast medium enhancement features for optimal characterisation of lesions. Not required for staging renal tumours.

- 100-150 ml of intravenous iodinated contrast medium injected at 3-4 ml/sec.

- MDCT with acquisition in the cortico-medullary phase at 30 seconds performed through the abdomen only. (This is of particular importance if considering nephron-sparing surgery in order to optimally visualise the arterial anatomy.)

- Post-contrast MDCT at 65 seconds from lung apices to iliac crest. This will allow opacification of renal veins and the IVC, as well as allowing visualisation of the primary tumour.

- For lesion characterisation (prior to definitive diagnosis), post-contrast MDCT should be performed at 80-100 seconds to provide a true nephrographic phase of enhancement.

- Using MDCT, slice thickness will depend on scanner capability. In general, sections are acquired at 1.25-2.5 mm and reformatted at 5 mm for viewing.

Values of $CTDI_{vol}$ should normally be below the relevant national reference dose for the region of scan and patient group (see Appendix and section on *Radiation Protection for the Patient in CT* in chapter 2).

MRI

MRI is used to solve problems, e.g., assess extent of venal caval invasion.

Protocol for imaging of anal canal cancer				
Sequence	Plane	Slice thickness	Field of view	Principle observations
T1W	Axial	6 ± 2 mm	Large	Primary tumour Venous invasion Lymph node involvement
T2W*	Axial	6 ± 2 mm	Large	
T1W + Fat Sat	Axial	6 ± 2 mm	Large	
T1W + Fat Sat (+C)	Axial	6 ± 2 mm	Large	
T1W	Sagittal / coronal	6 ± 2 mm	Large	Inferior vena cava and renal vein invasion

Respiratory triggering

Abdominal surface coil (torso) should be used whenever possible. Optional sequences include T1W with ECG gating if supradiaphragmatic extension is suspected. GRE T1W ± C as an option to Fat Sat T1 (above) to assess venous patency.

Suggested renal vein / caval protocol (additional)

3-D fat-saturated GRE sequence.

- At the onset of examination (0 seconds) 0.1 mmol/kg patient body weight gadolinium containing contrast medium mixed with 20 ml saline injected at 4 ml/sec with 20 seconds data acquisition at 20, 50 and 80 seconds post-injection.

PET-CT

[18]FDG PET-CT is not used for primary renal tumour assessment as [18]FDG is excreted in the urine and therefore uptake by tumour may be masked. Furthermore, primary renal cell carcinoma displays wide-ranging uptake of [18]FDG from negative through to intense. [18]FDG PET-CT is useful for the demonstration of metastatic disease, particularly for the demonstration of lytic metastatic bone disease. It is also useful for assessing response of bone metastases to treatment.

Follow-up

The frequency of follow-up depends on stage and histology at presentation at surgery. In principle, larger tumours with lymph node infiltration or venous tumour extension are reviewed more frequently. Data now suggest that no follow-up is needed for T1 N0 M0 tumours. Best available data suggest T2 and T3 tumours not receiving adjuvant therapy are scanned at 24 and 60 months or when symptomatic. Patients with T3a tumours are rescanned at 3-6 months following surgery.

CT is optimal technique. Only post-contrast scans to include chest and abdomen are required.

Tips

- Following nephrectomy, unopacified loops of small bowel dropping into the renal resection bed can cause confusion and bowel opacification is advised.

- As 30% of recurrent disease occurs in the chest, follow-up should always include imaging of the chest.

Adrenocortical cancer

Clinical background

Adrenocortical carcinomas are rare and only account for 0.05-0.2% of all cancers, have a bimodal age distribution (before 5 years of age and in the 4th-5th decades), and are often found to be "functioning" in children, where the majority present with virilization (40%) or in combination with Cushing's syndrome (50%). Prognosis is very poor; even in those undergoing complete resection, 85% will recur.

Who should be imaged?

All patients with a histologically diagnosed adrenocortical carcinoma should be staged.

Staging objectives

- To detect invasion of adjacent viscera.
- To identify venous invasion.
- To identify lymph node enlargement.
- To identify distant metastases.

Staging

CT

CT is the technique of choice.

- The abdomen and chest should be examined.
- Unenhanced scan through the abdomen.
- 100-150 ml of intravenous iodinated contrast medium injected at 3-4 ml/sec.
- MDCT with acquisition at 30 seconds through the abdomen.
- MDCT from lung apices to iliac crest at 65 seconds.
- Reformatting test images in sagittal and coronal planes allows optimal assessment of infiltration of adjacent viscera.
- Using MDCT, slice thickness will depend on scanner capability. In general, sections are acquired at 1.25-2.5 mm and reformatted at 5 mm for viewing.

Values of $CTDI_{vol}$ should normally be below the relevant national reference dose for the region of scan and patient group (see Appendix and section on *Radiation Protection for the Patient in CT* in chapter 2).

Follow-up

CT of the abdomen as a baseline following surgery and if relapse is suspected.

Tip

- MDCT reformatted images provide a useful vascular map prior to surgical resection.

Evaluation of the incidental adrenal gland mass in patients with cancer

Staging objectives

- To distinguish between adrenal adenomas and non-adenomatous masses in patients with cancer

CT

Adrenals

- Pre-contrast scan.

- Intravenous injection of 100 ml contrast medium at 3-4 ml/sec.

- Acquisition through the adrenals at 1 minute and 10 minutes.

- Using MDCT, slice thickness will depend on scanner capability. In general, sections are acquired at 1.25-2.5 mm and reformatted at 5 mm for viewing.

- Measure attenuation value on all scans using the longest ROI to fill the lesion.

Calculate contrast medium washout using the following formula: where
A_D = attenuation value at 10 min
A_U = attenuation of unenhanced image
A_1 = attenuation value at 1 min.

$$\frac{A_1 \ A_D}{A_1 \ A_U} \ x \ 100$$

A value of about greater than 60% is about 98% specific for an adrenal adenoma.

Values of $CTDI_{vol}$ should normally be below the relevant national reference dose for the region of scan and patient group (see Appendix and section on *Radiation Protection for the Patient in CT* in chapter 2).

MRI

Adrenals

- Spin-echo T1W sequence to localise adrenal glands.

- Gradient-recalled echo in-phase sequence (usually 4.2 msec at 1.5 Tesla).

- Gradient-recalled echo out-of-phase sequence.

Calculate signal intensity loss by evaluating the Signal Intensity Index (SII):

$$\frac{SI \ (in\text{-}phase) - SI \ (out\text{-}of\text{-}phase)}{SI \ (in\text{-}phase)} \quad x \quad \frac{100}{1}$$

A value exceeding SI (in-phase) >11.2% is >95% specific for an adenoma.

PET-CT

[18]FDG PET-CT is useful to differentiate benign from malignant adrenal lesions; adenomas do not demonstrate significant [18]FDG uptake whereas metastases are usually [18]FDG intense. The one caveat is that adrenal hyperplasia may show low to moderate grade [18]FDG uptake.

CHAPTER 13

Bladder cancer and other urothelial tumours

Clinical background

Bladder cancer is the commonest tumour of the urinary tract. It is usually a disease of the 6th and 7th decades, and the incidence is rising. More than 90% of tumours are transitional cell carcinomas (TCC) involving the lateral bladder walls and trigone; adenocarcinomas are often associated with a patent urachus. Approximately one-third of patients have multifocal disease at presentation, and the entire mucosa is considered as being unstable (that is, field changes are present). The latter is associated with an increased risk of developing invasive and recurrent disease.

Superficial, non-invasive bladder tumours may be treated with local therapy such as cystoscopic resection, diathermy, or intravesical chemotherapy. Invasive disease confined to the bladder wall or with minimal extravesical spread is suitable for treatment by cystectomy alone. However, with more advanced disease, combination treatment with chemotherapy and/or radiotherapy may be used to downstage disease prior to surgery, or with palliative intent.

Regional nodal spread is to the nodes of the true pelvis, i.e., the internal and external iliac groups. Nodal spread to the common iliac or retroperitoneal groups is regarded as metastatic.

Who should be imaged?

Once a diagnosis of invasive bladder cancer has been established from cystoscopic biopsy, the imaging modality for formal staging depends on treatment intent. If patients are considered suitable for radical treatment, MRI is the preferred modality. Where there is suspicion of locally advanced or metastatic disease precluding radical treatment, then CT is recommended.

Staging objectives

To identify evidence of:

- Full thickness mural involvement by tumour.
- Extent of extravesical tumour spread.

- Regional lymph node involvement.
- Metastatic adenopathy.
- Evidence of peritoneal dissemination of disease.

Staging

MRI is superior to CT for staging bladder cancer, due to its ability to demonstrate muscle wall invasion or penetration. Its multiplanar imaging capacity allows assessment of tumour involvement of adjacent organs. MRI is the imaging modality of choice for staging patients considered suitable for radical treatment, that is cystectomy or radical radiotherapy. In those patients who are not suitable for radical treatment or where there is clinical suspicion of locally advanced or metastatic disease, CT of the abdomen and pelvis is suitable of staging purposes.

MRI

MRI of the abdomen and pelvis should be performed.

T2W sequences give high contrast between tumour and intravesical urine whilst T1W images give sharp demarcation of the outer contour of the bladder against pelvic fat. Dynamic contrast-enhanced T1W fat saturated sequences demonstrate tumour, invasion and multifocality. Overview sequences of the pelvis and retroperitoneum assess for nodal metastases and hydronephrosis.

Protocol for imaging of bladder and other urothelial tumours				
Sequence	Plane	Slice thickness	Field of view	Principle observations
T1W	Axial whole pelvis	6 mm	Large	Nodal and bone assessment
T2W	Axial / coronal / sagittal – 2 of 3 orientations depending on tumour site	3.5 mm	Small	Primary tumour assessment
T1W gradient echo with fat suppression before and immediately after contrast medium	As above		Small (Scan immediately)	Depth of tumour invasion / transmural and extravesical spread
T2W	Axial		Large – abdomen and pelvis	Lymph nodes Hydronephrosis Ascites

CT

Contrast-enhanced images of the abdomen and pelvis are required to assess the primary tumour, its relationship to adjacent structures, and interrogation of the retroperitoneum and pelvis for adenopathy, and the liver for the presence of metastases.

- Oral administration of 1 litre of water as a contrast agent, of which 400 ml to be drunk immediately prior to going onto the scanner (see Tips).
- 100-150 ml of intravenous iodinated contrast medium injected at 3-4 ml/sec.

- MDCT is commenced at 70-80 seconds post-injection to assess the abdomen and pelvis.

- A maximum slice thickness of 5 mm is required using spiral technique.

- Using MDCT, slice thickness will depend on scanner capability. In general, sections are acquired at 1.25-2.5 mm and reformatted at 5 mm for viewing.

- For unusual histological tumour types such as small cell bladder cancers, scanning of the thorax should also be performed.

Values of $CTDI_{vol}$ should normally be below the relevant national reference dose for the region of scan and patient group (see Appendix and section on *Radiation Protection for the Patient in CT* in chapter 2).

PET-CT

^{18}FDG PET-CT is not useful for the assessment of bladder cancer and other urothelial tumours as the radiotracer is excreted within urine physiologically.

Follow-up

CT is the primary imaging modality for follow-up with the same protocol as above. Where combination therapy is used, timing of follow-up will be dictated by chemotherapy cycles and planned surgery. With primary surgical management, there is no clear evidence base to dictate frequency and duration of follow-up. Reassessment at 6 months and 1 year is often undertaken, subsequent imaging then depending on disease status and patient symptoms.

Tips

- An empty bladder should be avoided, as under such circumstances it is not possible to assess the primary tumour. For CT, the patient should be scanned with a full bladder for optimal assessment. Due to the time required for an MRI study, the bladder should not be full at the start of the examination to avoid movement artefact.

- A catheterised patient should have the catheter clamped prior to scanning.

- The site of the primary tumour within the bladder will determine the optimal imaging plane.

- For tumours involving the ureteric orifices, careful scrutiny of potential ureteric spread is important as this may alter management.

Upper urinary tract tumours

Clinical background

Upper tract transitional cell cancers (TCC) are usually suspected to be present following investigations of patients presenting with haematuria. A filling defect in the collecting system on intravenous urogram is the typical finding of TCC; ureteroscopy and biopsy are usually undertaken to confirm the diagnosis, and CT is then performed for staging the tumour. If ureteroscopy has been unsuccessful, CT is appropriate for further assessment. Nephroureterectomy is the treatment of choice for transitional tumours of the renal pelvis and ureters, either as the primary modality or in combination with chemotherapy where there is evidence of metastatic disease at staging.

Who should be imaged?

CT is recommended in all patients with suspected upper tract TCC for both diagnostic and staging purposes. MR urography is the modality of choice for imaging suspected lower ureteric tumours. The above recommendations apply regardless of treatment intent.

Staging objectives

- To identify the primary tumour site, its size and tumour extent.
- To identify if multifocal lesions are present.
- To detect nodal metastases.
- For surveillance of the remainder of the urinary tract.

Staging

Triple-phase (pre-, post- and delayed-contrast) contrast medium enhanced CT is the imaging modality of choice for the investigation and assessment of suspected urothelial tumours involving the pelvicalyceal systems and upper ureters. MR urography is indicated for the investigation and assessment of lower ureteric tumours.

CT

CT of the abdomen and pelvis should be performed. Contrast-enhanced images of the abdomen and pelvis allow assessment of enhancement within the suspected primary tumour, interrogation of the retroperitoneum and pelvis for lymphadenopathy and the liver for the presence of metastases.

The entire urothelial system to the bladder base should be imaged due to the risk of multiple lesions.

For upper urothelial tumours
- Oral administration of 1 litre of water as a contrast agent, of which 400 ml to be drunk immediately prior to going onto the scanner (see Tips).
- Unenhanced scans through the kidney and proximal ureters (depending on the level of lesion on IVU) are crucial to identify calculi or tumour surface calcium.
- 100-150 ml of intravenous iodinated contrast medium injected at 3-4 ml/sec.
- MDCT is commenced at 70-80 seconds post-injection to assess the abdomen and pelvis.
- A maximum slice thickness of 5 mm is required using spiral technique.
- Using MDCT, slice thickness will depend on scanner capability. In general, sections are acquired at 1.25-2.5 mm and reformatted at 5 mm for viewing.
- Delayed images through the kidneys and upper ureters aid in the identification of small tumours as filling defects within the opacified collecting system.

Values of CTDI$_{vol}$ should normally be below the relevant national reference dose for the region of scan and patient group (see Appendix and section on *Radiation Protection for the Patient in CT* in chapter 2).

MRI

For lower urothelial tumours

Anti-peristaltic agent may be helpful. An abdomino-pelvic surface coil should be used where available.

Sequence	Plane	Slice thickness	Field of view	Reason
T2W	Axial	8-10 mm	Large abdomen	Hydronephrosis and adenopathy
T2W	Axial	6-8 mm	Large pelvis	Tumour extent and relationships Nodal involvement
Heavily T2W fast spin-echo sequence	Coronal	Thick slab	large	Identify level of ureteric obstruction
T2W	Coronal-oblique	2 mm	Small through tumour	Assess primary tumour extent

85

Follow-up

CT is the primary imaging modality for follow-up after nephroureterectomy or where there is evidence of metastatic disease. In patients receiving systemic treatment for metastatic disease, the timing and frequency of reassessment is usually determined by chemotherapy schedules and planned surgery. For early stage disease treated with primary surgery, there is no clear evidence base for timing and frequency of follow-up, which is therefore often dictated by patient symptoms.

Tips

- It is essential to review the pre-contrast images to exclude calculous disease.
- The pyelogram-phase images are helpful to differentiate urothelial from renal cortical tumours.
- The thick slab HASTE sequence allows appropriate MR planning of the thin section T2W sequence through the lower ureteric tumour.

CHAPTER 14

Prostate cancer

Clinical background

Prostate cancer is the second commonest cause of male cancer death. An increasing incidence and patient awareness, together with technical developments in treatment, have generated an increased need to improve imaging to detect and stage the tumour initially, to help determine the most appropriate treatment for individual patients and to detect relapse disease after definitive therapy. Monitoring local disease response is not generally in the realm of imaging. Diagnosis is usually established on directed ultrasound-guided biopsy or as an incidental finding on histological reviews of chippings from transurethral resection of the prostate usually done for benign prostatic hyperplasia (BPH). Appropriate treatment selection for prostate cancer requires high quality and clinically relevant imaging that is best managed through urology MDT working, where diagnostic radiologists can understand underlying clinical issues and where clinicians can appreciate the indications for, limitations of and developments in imaging that are available to them. In the early 21st century, prostate imaging incorporates sophisticated and highly accurate anatomical imaging and physiological and biological imaging yielding an expanding volume of data about tumour extent.

The interpretation of imaging findings and clinical information determines the feasibility of radical treatments, either surgery or radiotherapy, or palliative therapy. Thus,

- If disease is organ-confined, radical treatment may be offered without adjuvant treatment.

- If disease is largely organ-confined with small volume periprostatic or seminal vesicle spread, radical radiotherapy can still be offered with / without pelvic nodal irradiation or with / without adjuvant hormonal therapy.

- The presence of suspected apical tumour will affect radiotherapy margins and alter the surgical approach with regard to the prostatic apex.

- Patients presenting with locally advanced or metastatic disease should not usually require detailed local tumour staging.

The choice of which imaging technique to use depends on the clinical presentation and the intent to treat actively or otherwise; elderly men with clinically insignificant prostate cancers may well not require any imaging at all. Such patients can be monitored with serum PSA (prostate-specific antigen) as necessary and medical intervention with hormonal therapy can usually be based on this without the need for cross-sectional imaging.

Who should be imaged?

The majority of urologists and urological radiologists agree that the following patient categories should be imaged using MRI: symptomatic patients as MRI has an important contributing role in determining tumour extent, detecting complications and planning treatment; patients at higher risk of local / metastatic spread with PSA greater than 12 ng/ml, Gleason score 8-10 and clinical stage T3 or T4; potential surgical candidates where Partin tables suggest the risk of extra-prostatic disease is greater than 45%; and patients with palpable apical tumours.

Staging objectives

- To delineate the intra- and extra-prostatic extent of the local disease. Here, the key distinction is organ confinement versus extra-prostatic disease. Prostatic cancer is often multifocal, and the detection of the dominant prostatic cancer nodule is becoming important for therapy planning.

- To detect the presence of cancer at the prostatic apex; this is an important consideration for a patient being considered for surgical therapy.

- To detect the presence and location (intra- versus extra-pelvic) of nodal enlargement.

- To detect the presence of bone metastases.

- To detect the presence of complications of urinary tract obstruction.

Staging

Currently, imaging on a 1.5 Tesla scanner is recommended with a surface pelvic-phased array coil. An endorectal coil may yield additional benefits due to increased signal-to-noise ratio and the ability to perform higher resolution imaging, but it cannot be recommended for all patients. Magnetic resonance spectroscopy (MRS) is best performed using endorectal coil acquisition. In the future, imaging at 3 Tesla may become standard and imaging protocols will need to be adapted.

MRI

MRI is the imaging technique of choice for clinically localised prostate cancer when radical treatment is under consideration. Radical surgery, radiotherapy or other forms of locally ablative therapy require accurate delineation of disease extent and the likely nodal status. However, it should be noted that MRI has a selective role for newly diagnosed cancers. A bowel relaxant may be used to improve quality of images.

Protocol for imaging of prostate tumours (at 1.5T)				
Sequence	Plane	Slice thickness	Field of view	Reason
TIW	Axial prostate	3 mm (max)	Small (e.g., 20 cm)	To detect the presence of intraprostatic blood and to delineate other outline of the gland
T2W	Axial prostate	3 mm	Small	Local staging, detection of dominant intraprostatic nodule and apical tumour
T2W	Coronal prostate	3 mm	Small	Local staging particularly involvement of prostatic base and adjacent seminal vesicle invasion. Nodal involvement also well shown
T2W-FSE	Axial abdomen (Breath-hold) & pelvis (non-breath-hold)	5-6 mm	Large	Nodal involvement Renal obstruction
T1W-SE	Axial pelvis	5-6 mm	Large	Nodal involvement and bone metastatic disease

T2W FSE sequences give the optimum contrast between tumour and normal prostate in the peripheral zone whilst T1W images give sharp demarcation of the outer contour of the prostate against periprostatic fat. The echo train length of FSE sequences should not be excessive (greater than 30) because image blurring will occur. Differentiation of tumour from nodular BPH in the central gland is difficult on all sequences.

Sagittal plane imaging does not usually contribute and is not recommended for routine use.

Dynamic contrast-enhanced T1W sequences may help to improve the localisation of the tumour within the gland; they have been shown to better demonstrate small volume extraprostatic disease extension (both T3A / T3B disease) and may have a role in planning brachytherapy seed / catheter placement and in planning intensity modulated radiotherapy (IMRT).

Magnetic resonance spectroscopy is now becoming commercially available and is likely to have a role in the pre-treatment assessment of patients for brachytherapy and IMRT. It may also have a role in the serial monitoring of patients who opt for active surveillance of their prostate cancer by monitoring metabolic activity (changes in tumour grade / aggressiveness may be reflected in spectroscopic appearances).

MR lymphography using ultra-small super-paramagnetic iron oxide particles (USPIOs) show promise for the nodal evaluation in patients with prostate malignancy. They are, as yet, not commercially available, and their initial role will be in patients with borderline nodal enlargement or those at high risk of nodal involvement with normal sized nodes on imaging where therapy would be altered by the detection of nodal disease.

CT

CT does not have a role in T-staging prostate cancer and is not recommended. The contribution of CT is in the assessment of nodal status and in detecting metastatic bone disease.

CT of the abdomen and pelvis should be performed.

- Oral administration of 1 litre of water or iodinated contrast medium.
- 100-150 ml of intravenous iodinated contrast medium injected at 3-4 ml/sec.
- MDCT is commenced at 70-80 seconds post-injection to assess the abdomen and pelvis.
- A maximum slice thickness of 5 mm is required using spiral technique.
- Using MDCT, slice thickness will depend on scanner capability. In general, sections are acquired at 1.25-2.5 mm and reformatted at 5 mm for viewing.

Values of $CTDI_{vol}$ should normally be below the relevant national reference dose for the region of scan and patient group (see Appendix and section on *Radiation Protection for the Patient in CT* in chapter 2).

Note: 99^mTc labelled MDP is superior to CT for detecting bone disease.

PET-CT

^{18}FDG PET-CT does not currently have a role in the staging of primary prostate cancer. Newer isotopes such as 11C-citrate and 11C-choline are in development, but their roles are incompletely defined.

Follow-up

Follow-up for prostate cancer will depend on the type of treatment used. Routine imaging follow-up is not indicated following radical treatment (either surgery or radiotherapy).

- Biochemical failure (serial rising serum PSA levels) may require imaging to try to determine whether the recurrence is confined to the pelvis (local) and / or systemic. Local salvage treatment which can be successful will require the exclusion, as far as possible, of distant metastases.
- MRI is more helpful than CT for assessing the prostate bed following radical prostatectomy. Dynamic contrast enhancement may be useful for differentiating scar tissue from active disease.
- Non contrast medium enhanced MRI is often unhelpful following radical prostate radiotherapy, and CT can be used since the only useful information is the possible identification of lymph node metastases.

Tips

- When reporting prostate MRI, it is useful to refer to Partin tables (http://urology.jhu.edu/Partin_tables/) which provide the pre-test probability of organ confinement, seminal vesicle invasion and nodal involvement. These tables are particularly helpful when imaging findings are equivocal and staging will affect treatment. It has been shown that this approach improves accuracy of staging overall.
- Prostatic haemorrhage is universally seen after transrectal biopsy of the prostate and can take many weeks to clear. The presence of haemorrhage can lead to an under- or over-estimate of the extent of intra-prostatic disease. Occasionally, blood can lead to blurring of the prostatic capsule making the evaluation of small volume extra-prostatic disease problematic. Caution should be exercised in interpreting minimal extra-prostatic spread in the presence of haemorrhage.

CHAPTER 15

Testicular cancer

Clinical background

95% of testicular cancers are of germ cell origin. Of these, 60% are non-seminomatous germ cell tumour (NSGCT, teratoma) and 40% are seminoma. Mixed germ cell tumours may occur and are treated as NSGCT. Testicular lymphoma, paratesticular rhabdomyosarcoma and a variety of rare tumours may also occur and are treated according to the histological origin of the primary. Orchidectomy is performed for most patients with NSGCT and pathological staging of the primary identifies risk factors for metastatic disease, such as lymphatic and vascular invasion. Germ cell tumours are frequently associated with raised serum markers; beta human chorionic gonadotrophin (β-HCG), and alpha-foetoprotein (AFP) estimations are important in diagnosis and follow-up.

The patterns of spread of testicular tumours are predictable. NSGCT typically spreads initially to the retroperitoneal lymph nodes, but pulmonary metastatic disease may be seen at first presentation. Seminoma metastasises to lymph nodes in the retroperitoneum, and eventually mediastinum, rarely involving lung and other organs.

Historically, a variety of staging systems have been used, many reliant on clinical assessment of mass lesions. The Royal Marsden Hospital (RMH) staging system for testicular tumours was developed at a time when improvements in body CT allowed identification of mediastinal and retroperitoneal lymph nodes and pulmonary deposits. The TNM system has been modified to resemble the RMH system but is not in uniform use.

Who should be imaged?

Following orchidectomy and an established diagnosis of a testicular germ cell tumour, all patients should be staged with CT. For NSGCT, this should include chest, abdomen and pelvis. Follow-up depends on disease stage at presentation, and some patients may be suitable for surveillance programmes (see over).

All patients with seminoma should be staged with CT of abdomen and pelvis at presentation. It is an option to include thoracic CT in the initial assessment, as the discovery of retroperitoneal nodal enlargement would necessitate thoracic CT

Staging objectives

- To detect lymph node metastases in abdomen, thorax and supraclavicular fossa.
- To identify lung metastases.
- To identify disseminated blood-borne metastatic disease, e.g., in the liver.
- To identify brain metastases in selected patients.

Note that the primary tumour is not assessed by CT or MRI.

Staging nodal and metastatic disease CT

CT is the preferred investigation, as it remains the most sensitive modality for identifying small (less than 1 cm) pulmonary metastases. For NSGCT, because of the relatively high incidence of chest deposits, CT scanning of whole body is preferred. At initial staging of all germ cell tumours contrast-enhanced CT of the thorax, abdomen and pelvis should be obtained although subsequently some body areas (e.g., pelvis) may be omitted particularly in patients who have had standard (that is, inguinal) orchidectomy. However, in patients who have had a scrotal incision, inguinal hernia repair, or developed testis cancer in an ectopic / undescended testis, the pelvis should be imaged on follow-up examinations.

- Oral administration of 1 litre of water or iodinated contrast medium.
- 100-150 ml of intravenous iodinated contrast medium injected at 3-4 ml/sec.
- MDCT is commenced at 25-30 seconds post-injection to assess the thorax and 70-80 seconds post-injection to assess the abdomen and pelvis.
- Alternative protocol for 16-slice MDCT: commence scanning at 50 seconds post-injection to include chest, abdomen and pelvis.
- A maximum slice thickness of 5 mm is required using spiral technique.
- Using MDCT, slice thickness will depend on scanner capability. In general, sections are acquired at 1.25-2.5 mm and reformatted at 5 mm for viewing.

Values of $CTDI_{vol}$ should normally be below the relevant national reference dose for the region of scan and patient group (see Appendix and section on *Radiation Protection for the Patient in CT* in chapter 2).

MRI

MRI has similar sensitivity to CT for detection of nodes in the retroperitoneum but in general is not used for this purpose. MRI is the technique of choice for detecting brain metastases. If a patient presents with more than 20 pulmonary metastases or HCG level greater than 10,000, brain deposits are sufficiently likely that MRI is indicated. The trophoblastic subtype of NSGCT is also associated with a high incidence of brain deposits. The brain may act as a "sanctuary site" for NSGCT deposits during treatment with chemotherapy.

Follow-up

Surveillance

Following orchidectomy for NSGCT, patients may be assigned Stage 1, if there is no distant spread on CT. Approximately 70% of Stage I patients will not relapse and can enter a surveillance programme which involves serum tumour marker estimations and regular CT follow-up. Of those patients with Stage I tumours who will relapse (30%), 80% will do so within 1 year, and 95% within 2 years. In general, follow-up surveillance CT makes no distinction between patients at high and low risk and is usually undertaken at 3-monthly intervals up to 12 months and 6-monthly intervals up to 2 years. Some centres opt for more intensive surveillance; that is: 3, 6, 9, 12 and 24 months. Imaging surveillance may then be discontinued and the patient followed clinically and with serum marker estimations.

Surveillance programmes are rarely used in seminoma. Relapse rates on surveillance are approximately 15%. Following radiation therapy to the retroperitoneum, the relapse rate falls to 1%, and this is the usual treatment pathway. If surveillance is undertaken for Stage 1 seminoma, scans at 6, 12, 24, 36, 48 and 60 months should be performed.

Rising tumour marker levels will usually precipitate further imaging to identify metastatic disease or a new primary tumour; this usually requires CT of chest, abdomen and pelvis together with ultrasound of the remaining testicle. If no new disease is seen, an MRI of the brain is also indicated as this may be a site of occult metastatic disease. [18]FDG PET-CT should also be considered, if available.

Follow-up for metastatic disease

Non-seminomatous germ cell tumours
CT should be performed using the same protocol as for staging, using intravenous contrast medium.

All sites of disease should be assessed according to response criteria and residual masses following completion of treatment and should be assessed for possible surgical excision in terms of size, precise location and relationship to adjacent structures, including major vessels. [18]FDG PET-CT is evolving as an important modality to identify residual active disease in patients with demonstrable residual masses.

Seminomas
In general seminomatous residual masses are not resected, because the majority comprise fibrosis and necrosis with no evidence of active residual malignancy.

Tips

- Brain metastases are haemorrhagic and are frequently clearly identified on pre-contrast scans using CT or MRI.

- Nodal metastases in non-seminomatous germ cell tumours may become cystic on treatment.

CHAPTER 16

Ovarian cancer

Clinical background

Ovarian cancer is the most frequent cause of death from gynaecological malignancy, and in the UK there were 6,884 new cases diagnosed in 1998. Neoplasms of surface epithelial origin account for 90% of malignant ovarian tumours, most commonly serous, followed by mucinous cystadenocarcinomas and endometrioid cancer. 60% of the serous tumours and 20% of the mucinous are bilateral. The majority occur between the ages of 30-40 years. Spread is by local extension, transcoelomic, and less commonly by the lymphatic and haematogenous routes. Transcoelomic spread occurs when the ovarian cancer breaks through the epithelial surface of the ovary and spills into the peritoneal cavity, and is most commonly seen in the omentum, the under surfaces of the diaphragm, surfaces of small and large bowel, surface of the liver, and the pouch of Douglas. Lymphatic drainage is via lymphatic channels accompanying the ovarian vessels: on the right these drain into the precaval and lateral caval lymph nodes between the right renal hilum and aortic bifurcation; on the left the lymph nodes are usually around the renal hilum.

Who should be imaged?

Patients with known ovarian cancer should be imaged using CT to assess degree of peritoneal involvement, particularly if chemotherapy is planned as a primary treatment. Patients presenting with peritoneal carcinomatosis should be imaged to assess the extent of disease, plan biopsy techniques, and assess other possible primary pathologies. CT is routinely used to monitor response to therapy and to detect recurrent disease. MRI is used to characterise indeterminate ovarian cysts or masses found on ultrasound, particularly in young patients or when CA -125 is normal or only slightly elevated.

Staging objectives

- To identify peritoneal involvement, particularly in the omenta, subphrenic spaces, falci form ligament, ascites, and serosal surfaces of small and large bowel.

- To determine involvement of pleural surfaces and pericardium.

- To detect lymph node enlargement, particularly in the retroperitoneum, paracardiac regions.

- To identify deposits in the liver and spleen.

- To identify urinary tract obstruction.

- Particularly in young or asymptomatic female patients in whom the CA-125 is normal or only mildly elevated, and ultrasound is indeterminate or positive for malignancy.

- To evaluate whether the ovarian pathology is benign or malignant.

- To decide pre-operatively whether cystectomy only is indicated or whether radical surgery is required.

Staging

- CT of the abdomen and pelvis should be performed to stage the primary tumour.

- CT is the most frequently used technique for staging ovarian cancer, but MRI is useful for characterising indeterminate ovarian pathology.

CT

- Oral administration of 1 litre of water as a contrast agent, of which 400 ml to be drunk immediately prior to going onto the scanner (see Tips).

- 100-150 ml of intravenous iodinated contrast medium injected at 3-4 ml/sec.

- MDCT is commenced at 70-80 seconds post-injection.

- Using MDCT, slice thickness will depend on scanner capability. In general, sections are acquired at 1.25-2.5 mm and reformatted at 5 mm for viewing.

Values of $CTDI_{vol}$ should normally be below the relevant national reference dose for the region of scan and patient group (see Appendix and section on *Radiation Protection for the Patient in CT* in chapter 2).

MRI

MRI of the pelvis. Bowel relaxant (buscopan or glucagons) may be helpful.

	Protocol for imaging of ovarian tumours				
Coils	Sequence	Plane	Slice thickness	Field of view	Principle observations
Abdomino-pelvic surface coil	T1W	Axial	6 ± 2 mm	Small (Pelvis + Abdomen)	Lymph nodes / Ascites Peritoneal / omental disease Hydronephrosis
	T2W	Axial	6 ± 2 mm	Small (Pelvis)	
	T2W	Sagittal	6 ± 2 mm	Large (Abdomen)	
	T1W T1 + Fat Sat	Axial	8 ± 2 mm	Small (Pelvis)	
	Dynamic contrast study T1 GRE	Axial	6 ± 2 mm	Small	To characterise small tumours
	T1 + Fat Sat	Axial	6 ± 2 mm	Small	
Liver (body coil may be used)	T2	Axial	6 ± 2 mm	Medium	Liver metastases
	T2	Coronal	6 ± 2 mm	Large (Cover abdomen: diaphragm to pubic symphysis)	To detect subphrenic spread

PET-CT

^{18}FDG PET-CT may be useful on occasion to define disease extent, particularly when follow-up surgery is being considered.

Follow-up

Follow-up is conducted:

- To assess response to chemotherapy and is therefore performed at a frequency to correspond with the chemotherapy regimes.

- To assess the need for and extent of interval debulking surgery.

- When there is marked evidence of recurrent disease (i.e., elevation of CA-125) and it is then performed to provide a baseline prior to chemotherapy.

- Prior to salvage surgery for isolated recurrences.

Tips

- On occasion, coronal or sagittal reformatted CT images may be very useful to distinguish between intrinsic liver and splenic lesions and peritoneal deposits in the subphrenic spaces.

- Water-filled bowel may allow better detection of serosal involvement than when filled with positive contrast agent.

- Peritoneal deposits are better demonstrated on contrast-enhanced GRE T1W sequences with fat suppression and are of value when ovarian pathology is characterised as malignant on MRI.

CHAPTER 17

96

Carcinoma of the cervix, vagina and vulva

Carcinoma of the cervix

Clinical background

The vast majority of cervical carcinomas are of squamous cell histology (85-90%); adenocarcinomas and adenosquamous carcinomas account for 10%. Cervical carcinoma spreads by direct tumour invasion through the stroma into the parametrium toward the pelvic wall. The uterosacral ligaments can also act as pathways of spread to the pelvic sidewall. Spread also occurs upward into the corpus of the uterus or downward into the vagina. Spread to the lymphovascular space extends to the paracervical, parametrial and presacral chains, and then the external iliac (obturator) internal iliac and common iliac nodes. Retroperitoneal and supraclavicular nodal involvement is only seen late in the course of the disease. Spread to the lungs, bone and liver is unusual. In large tumours, the key decision on imaging is to decide whether the parametrium is invaded, as this often determines the form of treatment. In young women, with small tumours who wish to retain the option to have children, consideration is given to a trachelectomy, conserving the uterus. Here, imaging must indicate the size of the tumour, its distance from the internal os, the length of the cervix, and the size of the uterus.

Who should be imaged?

All patients presenting with cytologically-proven cervical cancer, and to monitor response and detect recurrence in patients who have been treated with chemoradiotherapy.

Staging objectives

- To assess the size of the primary tumour.
- To identify the presence of parametrial spread.
- To identify proximal extension in relation towards the internal os, particularly in small tumours.

- To evaluate the pelvis and abdominal lymph nodes.
- To detect distant metastases.

Staging

MRI is the modality of choice, but CT is also a valuable technique for staging abdominal and pelvic disease.

MRI

Protocol for imaging of carcinoma of the cervix				
Sequence	Plane	Slice thickness	Field of view	Reason
T1W	Axial	6 ± 2 mm	Whole pelvis	To localise primary lesions or identify pelvic lymph nodes
T2W	Axial	6 ± 2 mm	Whole pelvis	
T2W	Sagittal	6 ± 2 mm	Small	
T2W Perpendicular to cervix	Oblique+	5 ± 2 mm	Small	To assess for parametrial spread
T1W / T2W	Coronal	6 ± 2 mm	Large	Abdominal lymph nodes and kidneys
T1W++	Axial	6 ± 2 mm	Medium / large (Abdomen)	

+ Perpendicular to plane of cervix and tumour
++ Optional: Performed if lymph node enlargement is identified in the pelvis

Pelvic-phased array coil is used. Intravenous bowel relaxants may be helpful for improving the quality of images by reducing motion artefact.

CT

- Oral administration of 1 litre of water or iodinated contrast medium.
- 100-150 ml of intravenous iodinated contrast medium injected at 3-4 ml/sec.
- MDCT is commenced at 60-75 seconds post-injection through the abdomen and pelvis.
- 5 mm axial sections using spiral technique.
- Using MDCT, slice thickness will depend on scanner capability. In general, sections are acquired at 1.25-2.5 mm and reformatted at 5 mm for viewing.

Values of $CTDI_{vol}$ should normally be below the relevant national reference dose for the region of scan and patient group (see Appendix and section on *Radiation Protection for the Patient in CT* in chapter 2).

PET-CT

[18]FDG PET-CT is not generally used in carcinoma of the cervix. On occasion, it may be helpful to define the presence and extent of metastases.

Follow-up

- Frequency depends on: form of treatment (surgical and / or radiotherapy) and size and histology of tumour at time of presentation.

- Following radiotherapy: MRI at 6 months, 1 year, and 2 years.

- Following surgery: MRI at 1 year, and 2 years.

Tips

- Care should be always be taken to ensure that the oblique axial T2 sequence is truly at right angles to the long axis of the cervix, otherwise mistakes can arise in interpreting parametrial invasion.

- Following intervention (such as a cone biopsy), changes can arise at the site of the biopsy that can be mistaken for the primary tumour. It is recommended that an interval of 1 week to 10 days be allowed between the biopsy and MRI.

- Occasionally, when the primary tumour remains poorly seen, dynamic contrast-enhanced scans in the sagittal plane may be used to better delineate tumour extent (as in endometrial cancer).

Carcinoma of the vagina and vulva

Clinical background

Primary vaginal cancer is rare. 85% are squamous cell occurring in the upper vagina in post-menopausal, often elderly women. About 5-10% are adenocarcinomas, 2-3% leiomyosarcomas, and 2-3% melanomas. Superficial carcinomas at the vaginal vault are treated by vaginectomy and pelvic lymphadenectomy. Tumours of the lower third of the vagina are usually treated by vulvectomy and inguinal lymphadenectomy.

Who should be imaged?

All patients who present with histologically-proven carcinoma of the vagina or vulva.

Staging objectives

- To identify nodal disease in the pelvis and inguinal regions.

- To determine the extent of the primary tumour.

- To identify intra-abdominal spread.

Staging

MRI

Protocol for imaging of liver metastases				
Sequence	Plane	Slice thickness	Field of view	Reasons
T1W	Axial	6 ± 2 mm	Whole pelvis & perineum *	To localise primary lesions or identify pelvic lymph nodes
T2W	Axial	6 ± 2 mm	Whole pelvis & perineum	
STIR	Axial	6 ± 2 mm	Perineum	Particularly to identify vulval tumours and inguinal nodes
T1W	Axial	6 ± 2 mm	Medium / large (Abdomen)	

* particularly for tumours of lower third.

Follow-up

If there is suspicion of clinical recurrence.

99

Tips

- Care should be taken to include the entire perineum, inguinal and femoral regions to ensure that all possible sites of infiltration and nodal involvement are included.

- For low vaginal and vulval tumours, ultrasound with fine needle aspiration biopsy may be extremely valuable in planning the lymph node dissection.

CHAPTER 18

Endometrial cancer

Clinical background

In the UK, the incidence of endometrial cancer is 4,900 per annum. 90% arise within the uterine epithelium and, of these, 90% are well-differentiated (Grade 1). The depth of myometrial invasion and invasion of the cervix stroma are the most important prognostic factors, e.g., the incidence of nodal metastases increases from 3% for Stage 1B (less than 50% myometrial invasion) to 40% for Stage 1C (greater than 50% myometrial invasion). Hence, staging of the tumour is crucial in deciding whether lymphadenectomy is indicated. Lymphadenectomy is a procedure that carries significant post-operative complications such as neuronal injury. Demonstration of cervical involvement may also determine that a radical rather than a simple hysterectomy is undertaken.

Who should be imaged?

At present, indications for MRI of the endometrium are not firmly established due to differing surgical practice with respect to lymphadenectomy. Nevertheless, there is general consensus that all patients with histological high-grade tumours should undergo MRI pre-operatively. In some centres all patients with histologically-proven endometrial carcinoma are scanned to identify patients with deep myometrial invasion or cervical involvement who would then be candidates for lymphadenectomy at surgery.

Staging objectives

- To identify whether there is myometrial invasion and, if so, to determine its depth (i.e., whether greater than 50% of myometrial thickness).

- To assess whether the tumour has spread outside the body of the uterus into the endocervical mucosa or into the cervical stroma.

- To identify whether the tumour has spread into the parametrium or the serosa.

- To identify lymph node enlargement. (Note: retroperitoneal nodes are considered regional.)

- To identify distant spread.

Staging

MRI is the technique of choice to stage the primary tumour within the pelvis, but CT is also a valuable technique for staging abdominal and pelvic disease.

Protocol for imaging of endometrial cancer				
Sequence	Plane	Slice thickness	Field of view	Reason
T2W	Sagittal (SE)	5 ± 2 mm	Whole pelvis	
T2W	Axial (SE)	5 ± 2 mm	Whole pelvis	
T2W	Oblique axial (SE) (perpendicular to long axis of uterus)	5 ± 2 mm	Small	To view the relationship between the primary tumour and the myometrium in a second plane
T1W + Fat Sat	Sagittal (GRE) Oblique axial	5 ± 2 mm		To optimise the assessment of the possibility of myometrial invasion
T1W + Fat Sat + IV contrast medium at 60 and 180 sec	Sagittal			
T1 + Fat Sat + IV contrast medium	Oblique axial		Small	
T1W	Axial	5 ± 2 mm	Standard	Mid-renal hilum to lymph node staging
T1W	Axial	6 ± 2 mm	Medium / large (Abdomen)	

Pelvic phased array coil is used. Intravenous bowel relaxants may be helpful for improving the quality of images by reducing motion artefact.

CT

- Oral administration of 1 litre of water or iodinated contrast medium.

- 100-150 ml of intravenous iodinated contrast medium injected at 3-4 ml/sec.

- MDCT is commenced at 60-75 seconds post-injection through the abdomen and pelvis.

- 5 mm axial sections using spiral technique.

- Using MDCT, slice thickness will depend on scanner capability. In general, sections are acquired at 1.25-2.5 mm and reformatted at 5 mm for viewing.

Values of $CTDI_{vol}$ should normally be below the relevant national reference dose for the region of scan and patient group (see Appendix and section on *Radiation Protection for the Patient in CT* in chapter 2).

Follow-up

- Frequency: Depends on the stage and histology of the disease at presentation. More advanced disease of higher grade histology is reviewed every 6 months following surgery, for up to 2 years. If treated only with radiotherapy, then follow-up is to assess response.

- Technique: MRI optimal modality of choice. Technique is modified and in general will include only:

  - Sagittal and axial spin-echo T2W sequences through the pelvis.

  - Axial or coronal SE or GRE T2W sequences through the abdomen.

Tip

- Data suggest that overall no significant statistical difference exists between T2W and contrast-enhanced sequences in predicting myometrial invasion. However, it is agreed that the 2 sequences are necessary to optimise accuracy and ease interpretation, particularly when uterine distortion is present (e.g., due to congenital abnormality of the uterus or due to fibroids). As the sensitivity for prediction of extension beyond the endometrium is the most important diagnostic parameter, it is better to rely on that sequence which indicates the most extensive disease.

CHAPTER 19

Lymphoma

Clinical background

Lymphoid malignancy is a diverse group of disorders derived from B-cells, T-cells and NK-cells that have a wide range of presentations, clinical course and response to therapy. Lymphoid neoplasms that present with masses are called lymphomas; those that have predominantly circulating cells are now termed leukaemias; those with both masses and circulating cells are called lymphoma / leukaemia. The incidence of Non-Hodgkin's lymphoma (NHL) has increased rapidly over the last few decades, while the incidence of Hodgkin's lymphoma (HL) is stable.

HL usually presents with lymphadenopathy in 1 or 2 contiguous sites. Untreated, it progresses with involvement of adjacent nodal sites and the spleen, before bone marrow, liver or lung involvement. NHL is divided into high- and low-grade. High-grade NHL often involves extra-nodal sites, such as the gastrointestinal or upper respiratory tract. It may spread to involve adjacent nodes, the liver, bone marrow or CNS. Low-grade NHL usually presents with generalised lymphadenopathy, with marrow and extra-nodal sites frequently involved.

The Ann Arbor classification is used for the anatomical staging for both HL and NHL, although there are potential problems with its NHL use. The TNM classification has adopted it for staging disease. Note that for the purposes of classification, lymph node, Waldeyer's ring and splenic involvement are considered nodal or lymphatic sites, and other organ involvement is considered extra-nodal.

Who should be imaged?

All patients with lymphoma, except perhaps those with limited cutaneous T-cell lymphoma, should be imaged for staging.

Staging objectives

- To stage nodal disease.
- To stage extra-nodal disease.
- To stage primary cerebral, orbital and head and neck lymphoma.
- To investigate suspected spinal cord compression.
- To assess marrow involvement.
- To evaluate musculoskeletal involvement.

Staging

CT is used as the main staging technique, with MRI used for well-defined clinical situations. Gallium scanning is used to provide functional imaging but is being replaced by ^{18}FDG PET-CT where available (see below for further ^{18}FDG PET-CT considerations).

CT

Routine staging should include the chest, abdomen and pelvis.

- Post-contrast medium scans through the chest and upper abdomen to include the liver and adrenal glands.
- 100-150 ml of intravenous iodinated contrast medium injected at 3-4 ml/sec.
- MDCT is commenced at 60-70 seconds to visualise optimally the liver in the portal venous phase and the intra-abdominal organs in the parenchymal phase of enhancement.
- If the neck is to be included the neck should be scanned at 25/30 seconds followed by the chest and abdomen.
- Using MDCT, slice thickness will depend on scanner capability. In general, sections are acquired at 1.25-2.5 mm and reformatted at 5 mm for viewing.

Note: Concerning the use of oral contrast medium, special attention should be paid to the bowel in NHL and positive contrast may be helpful.

Values of CTDI$_{vol}$ should normally be below the relevant national reference dose for the region of scan and patient group (see Appendix and section on *Radiation Protection for the Patient in CT* in chapter 2).

MRI

MRI is the investigation of choice for suspected CNS, musculoskeletal and marrow involvement. It may also be the initial investigation of choice in children and is used if the CT is equivocal. MRI protocols for individual areas are covered in the other chapters.

PET-CT

^{18}FDG PET-CT has replaced gallium scans for the assessment of metabolically active disease. ^{18}FDG PET-CT can identify disease in normal sized lymph nodes and at extra-nodal disease sites for both HL and NHL. It is not usually undertaken in low-grade NHL, unless the patient is going to be treated with radiotherapy when a single site of disease is identified. Mucosa-Associated Lymphoid Tissue (MALT) and mantle lymphoma have variable activity and may not demonstrate hypermetabolism.

^{18}FDG PET-CT can be used initially to stage the disease extent and may be used to assess effectiveness of therapy. ^{18}FDG PET-CT can be used for early assessment of response to treatment after 2 cycles of chemotherapy or at the end of treatment to confirm response. It can also be used to identify whether metabolically active disease is present in residual masses. It is recommended that at least 6 weeks should elapse between completion of therapy and ^{18}FDG PET-CT scanning. ^{18}FDG PET-CT should also be used to identify relapse when anatomical imaging is equivocal.

The widespread introduction of ^{18}FDG PET-CT in the UK may alter the staging investigations of lymphoma because of its potential to both stage and to follow treatment response in a single investigation.

Follow-up

Imaging objectives

- To assess response to treatment.
- To define the site and extent of residual masses and suspected recurrent disease.
- To follow-up both treated and untreated patients.

Follow-up imaging should be undertaken at 3 months after completion of therapy. Some institutions then undertake a scan at 6 months and 1 year, although other units will only scan at 3 months and 1 year. Either CT or MRI can be used, depending on the method used for the initial staging.

Evaluation of residual masses

CT is of limited value for evaluating the activity of residual disease. MRI is better at differentiating fibrosis from active disease based on signal characteristics, although MRI cannot always differentiate between early fibrosis and active disease. Current evidence suggests that ^{18}FDG PET-CT may be the best imaging technique for making this distinction.

CHAPTER 20

Musculoskeletal tumours

Primary bone tumours

Clinical background

Primary bone tumours are rare, but represent a widely diverse group of neoplasms. Virtually any connective tissue elements found in bone can undergo malignant change. The common bone tumours in young people are osteosarcoma, primitive neuroectodermal tumour, and Ewing's sarcoma. In older patients, chondrosarcoma, fibrosarcoma and chordoma are more common. There is also a wide variety of bone lesions which are non-malignant, such as chondroma, osteoid osteoma, non-ossifying fibroma, simple and aneurysmal bone cyst and Langerhans' cell histiocytosis. Plain film radiography is the most useful investigation for differential diagnosis. Any bone can be involved, but the distribution within the skeleton is an important factor in differential diagnosis. Biopsy is necessary to make a firm diagnosis of bone malignancy.

Who should be imaged?

All patients should be imaged at presentation to assess the extent of disease within the bone and soft tissues. Ideally this is performed before biopsy when a strong clinical suspicion of a primary bone tumour exists. Failing this, local staging may be performed following biopsy. All patients should have unenhanced thoracic CT at presentation.

Staging objectives

- To detect extent of bone marrow involvement, including involvement of the growth plate and skip lesions within the same bone.

- To detect the presence and extent of extraosseous soft tissue mass. These may extend into joint spaces and involve adjacent neurovascular bundles.

- To plan the optimal site and route for biopsy.

- To establish feasibility of surgical resection and design of endoprosthesis if indicated.

- To identify regional lymph node involvement.

- To assess for haematogenous metastatic spread, more frequently to the lung, but occasionally to other bones.

Staging

For primary diagnosis, plain radiographs should be used. For staging of local disease, MRI is the technique of choice, although contrast-enhanced CT can be employed. A local surface coil should be used if the tumour is not too large. Placement of skin surface markers may be useful.

Protocol for imaging of primary bone tumours				
Sequence	Plane	Slice thickness	Field of view	Reason
T1W	Sagittal / Coronal	5 ± 2 mm	To cover lesion	To show full extent of bone marrow involvement and skip lesions. Whole bone should be imaged including joints at both ends in long bones
T2W / STIR	Sagittal / Coronal	5 ± 2 mm	To cover lesion	To show full extent of bone marrow involvement and skip lesions. Whole bone should be imaged including joints at both ends in long bones
T2W	Axial	8 ± 2 mm	To cover lesion	To assess size of mass, compartmental involvement in limbs and proximity to neurovascular bundles
T1W	Axial	8 ± 2 mm	To cover lesion	
T1W gadolinium-enhanced	Axial or best plane to demonstrate anatomy	8 ± 2 mm	To cover lesion	To demonstrate enhancement patterns. Dynamic studies may be used.

Note: caution should be used interpreting STIR sequence, as it may overestimate extent of disease. Reactive oedema in bone and soft tissue can return abnormal signal on STIR sequence, and T1W and T2W imaging should be used to confirm disease extent. Use of contrast enhancement is not mandatory, but many radiologists prefer to use enhanced sequences with fat suppression to demonstrate extent of soft tissue masses.

CT

CT is recommended in all patients at diagnosis for assessment of pulmonary metastatic disease. If thoracic CT is normal at presentation, CXR may be used in follow-up. Follow-up for osteosarcoma entails more frequent use of chest CT, in particular, to follow previously demonstrated metastases, after thoracotomy or when new lesions are seen on CXR. For evaluation of regional nodal disease, ultrasound is the preferred technique in children. In the presence of bone pain elsewhere in the skeleton in patients with tumours, such as Ewing's sarcoma and osteosarcoma which are known to metastasise to other bones, isotope bone scan is the initial investigation.

Values of CTDI$_{vol}$ should normally be below the relevant national reference dose for the region of scan and patient group (see Appendix and section on *Radiation Protection for the Patient in CT* in chapter 2).

PET-CT

^{18}FDG PET-CT has a variable efficacy in sarcomas, depending on the tumour type and grade. The appearances range from very low-grade ^{18}FDG uptake through to intense uptake. ^{18}FDG PET-CT can be a useful modality for staging the extent of overall disease, particularly in primary tumours showing intense ^{18}FDG uptake, when surgery is being considered.

Follow-up

Neoadjuvant chemotherapy is routinely used for most bone sarcomas. Follow-up MRI using a technique similar to that employed at initial staging is carried out pre-operatively. Soft tissue masses are usually reduced in bulk by chemotherapy, and pathological evidence of necrosis in greater than 90% of the tumour implies a good prognosis. MRI can predict to some extent the expected degree of necrosis but is not entirely reliable. Marrow signal frequently remains abnormal, but prediction of histology from the residual abnormality is not possible. Granulocyte colony stimulating factor (G-CSF) is sometimes administered to prevent neutropenic sepsis, and regenerating islands of bone marrow may cause new areas of apparent abnormal MRI signal in the affected bone and elsewhere which should be interpreted with caution. Bone metastases are very unlikely to develop during neoadjuvant chemotherapy.

A baseline MRI 3 to 6 months after surgical resection is useful. Further follow-up depends on clinical suspicion for local recurrence, which in turn depends on histological features of the resected tumour. Surveillance for metastatic disease is also guided by clinical suspicion. Follow-up CXR is usually carried out regularly for up to 5 years.

Tips

- When staging primary bone tumours with MRI, skip lesions within the same bone should be actively sought.
- The STIR sequence may overestimate the extent of disease within the marrow in primary bone neoplasms.

Metastatic bone tumours

Clinical background

Bone metastases can be seen with any extracranial primary cancer. They are most frequently seen in patients with breast and prostate cancer, but lung, kidney, thyroid and gastrointestinal primaries frequently metastasise to bone. The initial investigation is usually isotope bone scan with confirmation by radiography, but MRI is slightly more sensitive in detection of metastatic bone disease. Isotope studies have the advantage of imaging the entire skeleton, but if patients have symptoms suggestive of metastatic bone disease, even with a normal bone scan and radiography, bone disease can still be documented by MRI.

Treatment of metastatic bone disease depends on the pathology of the primary tumour, and the number and distribution of lesions within the skeleton. Radiotherapy, chemotherapy and surgery may all be used in management of secondary bone deposits.

The majority of bone metastases develop in the same distribution as red marrow, with the spine in the lumbar region being most frequently affected. Pelvis, upper femora, upper humeri and skull vault are also commonly affected, but the more peripheral bones are unusual sites for bone metastases.

Who should be imaged?

Patients with suspected metastatic disease to bone should be selected for imaging on clinical grounds, taking into account the nature of the primary tumour and the length and severity of symptoms such as pain. These factors give an index of suspicion which helps to select patients for further investigation and, in turn, a high index of suspicion will lead to more intensive imaging investigation.

Imaging objectives

- To detect metastatic disease, define the number of metastases and extent within the same or other bones, and to demonstrate extent of soft tissue involvement.

- To detect actual or imminent epidural spinal cord compression by spinal lesions.

- To detect extent of bone disease at sites of high risk for fracture such as the femoral neck.

- To distinguish between metastatic and osteoporotic causes of vertebral collapse.

Imaging

MRI

This depends on the site of suspected abnormality. T1W sequences oriented to the bone or bones to be imaged will detect the majority of bone metastases. Metastatic tumour is of identical signal intensity to muscle and contrasts well with fat in the marrow cavity. In the spine, islands of residual red marrow can lead to diagnostic difficulty, but normal marrow distribution will be the same in each of the vertebral bodies. If there is doubt on the T1W sequence, the STIR sequence is helpful in highlighting pathology particularly in the dorsal elements. On T2W sequences, a tumour can be close to the signal of normal fatty marrow, and gadolinium enhancement on T1-weighted sequences reduces tumour to marrow contrast. Occasional gradient echo T2*W sequences, contrast medium enhancement and diffusion weighted images can be used to differentiate malignant from osteoporotic vertebral collapse.

CT

Reformatted MDCT spinal and pelvic images should be reviewed in the coronal and sagittal planes in patients with suspected bone metastases and in those with widespread soft tissue disease with primary tumours with a predilection to spread to bone (e.g., breast).

- Using MDCT, slice thickness will depend on scanner capability. In general, sections are acquired at 1.25-2.5 mm and reformatted at 5 mm for viewing.

Values of CTDI$_{vol}$ should normally be below the relevant national reference dose for the region of scan and patient group (see Appendix and section on *Radiation Protection for the Patient in CT* in chapter 2).

PET-CT

[18]FDG PET-CT is a particularly useful modality for the detection of metastatic bone disease being more specific than bone scan (uptake on PET represents uptake of tracer by active tumour cells whereas MDP bone scintigraphy demonstrates an osteoblastic response). [18]FDG PET-CT has the advantage of being able to demonstrate lytic bone metastases (which may not be demonstrated on bone scintigraphy) and a particularly promising area for [18]FDG PET-CT is in the evaluation of treatment response of metastatic bone disease.

Tip

- When bone metastases are suspected, bone scintigraphy is slightly less sensitive for detection of marrow disease than MRI, but isotope studies cover the whole skeleton.

Soft tissue sarcomas

Clinical background

These rare tumours represent a heterogeneous group of neoplasms with a wide spectrum of histological and clinical features. Most primary sarcomas are treated by surgery, but some such as rhabdomyosarcoma are treated with neoadjuvant chemotherapy followed by surgery if technically feasible. Sarcomas which cannot be completely resected may be treated with adjuvant radiotherapy. MRI is the investigation of choice for demonstration of extent of soft tissue tumours owing to its improved contrast resolution. Contrast medium enhanced CT may be substituted when MRI is not available or is contraindicated.

Who should be imaged?

All patients with suspected soft tissue sarcoma should have imaging staging of the primary tumour, preferably prior to biopsy. Once the diagnosis is established, all patients should have thoracic CT to stage for lung metastases. In certain tumour types, such as rhabdomyosarcoma of the lower limb or pelvis, abdominopelvic CT should be undertaken for nodal staging.

Staging objectives

- To identify the site and extent of soft tissue tumour.
- To plan biopsy.
- To define spread within muscle compartments and feasibility of resection.
- To identify regional lymph node metastases.

Staging

MRI

Surface coils or local coils should be used, where possible, if the tumour is not too large. Skin markers over palpable lesions are useful. T2W sequences yield the best contrast resolution, with tumour shown as high signal intensity when compared to adjacent muscle. T1W sequences are useful in the limbs to demonstrate any penetration into adjacent bone marrow.

Protocol for imaging of soft tissue sarcomas			
Sequence	Plane	Slice thickness	Field of view
T1W	Sagittal / Coronal	6 ± 2 mm	To cover lesion
T2W	Sagittal / Coronal	6 ± 2 mm	To cover lesion
T2 & T1W	Axial	8 ± 2 mm	To cover lesion
STIR	Best plane	8 ± 2 mm	To cover lesion
T1W with contrast medium enhancement	Best plane	8 ± 2 mm	To cover lesion

Footnote: STIR *sequence is useful to highlight pathology but may over estimate size of lesion*

CT

CT of thorax should be carried out at the time of diagnosis to detect pulmonary metastases. CXR should be performed at intervals in follow-up, depending on tumour biology.

- Using MDCT, slice thickness will depend on scanner capability. In general, sections are acquired at 1.25-2.5 mm and reformatted at 5 mm for viewing.

Values of $CTDI_{vol}$ should normally be below the relevant national reference dose for the region of scan and patient group (see Appendix and section on *Radiation Protection for the Patient in CT* in chapter 2).

PET-CT

Soft tissue sarcomas demonstrate a variable appearance with [18]FDG PET-CT, ranging from very low-grade through to intense uptake depending on the histological type and grade. In tumours which demonstrate intense [18]FDG uptake, the technique can be particularly useful for defining the overall extent of disease prior to surgery. Pulmonary nodules less than 7-10 mm in diameter may not be resolved on the PET component of current PET-CT technology.

Follow-up

Following surgical resection, MRI is a valuable technique for identifying recurrence. A baseline follow-up 6 months after surgery is useful, particularly if tumour was close to or involving resection margins. Skin markers placed at the extents of the surgical scar are helpful. Axial T2W sequences through the lesion will identify many tumours, but in follow-up examinations contrast medium enhancement is required to clarify any areas of abnormal signal intensity identified on T2W imaging. Any enhancing lesion with mass effect will require repeat biopsy or further surgery.

Tip

- Thoracic CT should be undertaken in patients with soft tissue sarcomas to identify pulmonary metastases.

CHAPTER 21

Paediatric neoplasms

Children's tumours are most appropriately imaged in centres where treatments will be given. Techniques and protocols should be according to patterns of tumour spread. An approach that obtains all the essential information at a single investigation is required if general anaesthetic or sedation are to be used. This should also include non-imaging investigations, such as bone marrow biopsy. In paediatric oncology, the TNM classification is not used. Alternative individual staging systems of common paediatric neoplasms (Wilms' tumour, neuroblastoma and rhabdomyosarcoma) are not included in this document.

Wilms' tumour

Clinical background

Wilms' tumour is the most frequent renal tumour of childhood and typically presents in the first 6 years of life with a painless abdominal mass. Initial imaging is usually with ultrasound, and the differential diagnosis includes nephroblastomatosis, clear cell sarcoma, renal cell carcinoma, renal lymphoma, and congenital mesoblastic nephroma. Tumours may be sufficiently large that the organ of origin is not always clear, and CT and MRI may be useful for discriminating between renal and adrenal mass lesions.

Who should be imaged?

All children presenting with an abdominal mass should be imaged initially with ultrasound. If Wilms' tumour is suspected or confirmed by biopsy, the primary tumour should be staged using CT or MRI.

Staging objectives

- To confirm the organ of origin.
- To assess tumour extent.

- To assess tumour extension into vessels.

- To detect local and regional lymph node involvement.

- To detect contralateral renal tumour.

- To detect distant metastatic disease (e.g., liver and lungs).

Staging

CT or MRI are used for assessment of abdominal disease. Ultrasound is the optimum method of assessing for tumour thrombus in the renal vein or inferior vena cava (IVC).

- With CT and MRI, IV contrast medium administration is mandatory to assess the primary tumour and contra-lateral kidney.

- Dosage of IV contrast medium is 1 ml/0.5 kg patient body weight with scanning at 65-70 seconds post-injection to allow opacification of renal veins and the IVC.

- Using MDCT, slice thickness will depend on scanner capability. In general, sections are acquired at 1.25-2.5 mm and reformatted at 5 mm for viewing.

Use of sedation or general anaesthesia depends on individual patient requirements and local circumstances.

113

CT of the chest may also be carried out at the same examination as staging of the primary tumour, although most international paediatric Wilms' studies rely solely on the findings on CXR to document pulmonary metastatic disease. CT or MRI can detect nodal and hepatic metastases and contralateral renal tumour. Ultrasound is helpful in detecting extension into vessels and direct involvement of liver.

Values of $CTDI_{vol}$ should normally be below the relevant national reference dose for the region of scan and patient group (see Appendix and section on *Radiation Protection for the Patient in CT* in chapter 2).

MRI

MRI technique is based on T2W and T1W spin-echo sequences in axial and coronal planes using a surface coil. Vascular supply and venous drainage may be assessed using angiographic sequences with / without IV contrast agents. A suggested protocol is as follows:

Protocol for imaging of Wilms' tumours			
Sequence	Plane	Slice thickness	Field of view
T1W	Axial	6 ± 2 mm	To fit patient
T2W	Axial	6 ± 2 mm	To fit patient
T1W	Coronal	6 ± 2 mm	To fit patient
T2W	Coronal	6 ± 2 mm	To fit patient
MR angiography or venography	3-D Coronal		To fit patient

Partial nephrectomy and other forms of nephron-sparing surgery are sometimes considered, particularly in the presence of bilateral tumours. Under these circumstances, angiographic studies may be of benefit to the surgeon.

Follow-up

Neoadjuvant chemotherapy is used initially for Wilms' tumour. Serial measurement with ultrasound is undertaken, often with a CT scan prior to surgical excision. Over 80% of Wilms' tumour relapses occur within 2 years after surgery. Following removal of the tumour, 3-monthly CXR and ultrasound examinations are employed initially; CT and MRI are not routinely employed in follow-up care.

Tips

- Post-contrast scans may demonstrate the normal renal cortex as a "claw" around the tumour.

- In patients with large tumour masses, nodal disease may be difficult to distinguish from the primary tumour.

Neuroblastoma

Clinical background

Neuroblastoma arises from cells of the embryonal neural crest, and there is a spectrum of disease that ranges from malignant undifferentiated neuroblastoma to well-differentiated ganglioneuroma. These tumours arise along the sympathetic neural axis, with the most frequent site being the adrenal glands. However, pelvic, thoracic and cervical neuroblastomas are also encountered. Peak age incidence is around 2 years. Surgery alone is adequate treatment for localised neuroblastoma, but the majority of patients present with more widespread tumour. Children over 1 year of age with an abdominal primary tumour often have metastatic disease at presentation (approx. 75%). Neuroblastoma diagnosed antenatally or in the first year of life behaves differently from tumours presenting later in childhood and has a good long-term prognosis.

Who should be imaged?

All patients with an abdominal mass or symptoms and signs suggestive of neuroblastoma should be imaged initially with abdominal ultrasound. Once the diagnosis of neuroblastoma is strongly suspected or confirmed, radionuclide imaging with metaiodobenzylguanidine (MIBG) should be undertaken in all patients. CT or MRI is used to stage the primary tumour (which may be extra-abdominal).

Staging objectives

- To characterise primary tumour and define extent.
- To identify encasement of vessels.
- To identify extension of tumour into spinal canal ('dumbbell' tumour).
- To identify bone erosion by primary tumour.
- To identify regional lymph node enlargement.
- To identify metastatic bone disease.

Staging

Ultrasound is frequently used as a first diagnostic investigation. MRI and CT can be used for staging of neuroblastoma. Radionuclide scanning with metaiodobenzylguanidine (MIBG) is performed routinely in all patients at diagnosis, and during follow-up in those with metastatic disease.

MRI

MRI is superior at diagnosing intra-spinal extension and metastatic disease in the bone marrow. Both techniques may be used and the choice is usually governed by availability of equipment.

Coil	Sequence	Plane	Slice thickness	Field of view
Protocol for imaging of neuroblastoma				
To fit patient	T1W	Axial	6 ± 2 mm	To fit patient
To fit patient	T2W	Axial	6 ± 2 mm	To fit patient
To fit patient	T1W	Coronal	6 ± 2 mm	To fit patient
To fit patient	T2W	Coronal	6 ± 2 mm	To fit patient
To fit patient	T1W + IV contrast medium MR angiography or venography	Axial / Coronal if required 3-D acquisition		To fit patient or body part

CT

MDCT is preferred, as reformatted images provide additional information useful for surgical planning.

- Dosage of IV contrast medium is 1 ml/0.5 kg patient body weight with scanning at 65-70 seconds post-injection to demonstrate arterial and venous anatomy.

- Using MDCT, slice thickness will depend on scanner capability. In general, sections are acquired at 1.25-2.5 mm and reformatted at 5 mm for viewing.

Values of $CTDI_{vol}$ should normally be below the relevant national reference dose for the region of scan and patient group (see Appendix and section on *Radiation Protection for the Patient in CT* in chapter 2).

Follow-up

Neoadjuvant chemotherapy is used to reduce tumour bulk, and repeat imaging prior to an attempt at surgical resection should use the same technique as at diagnosis. Post-surgical imaging is often undertaken to provide a baseline for follow-up. Subsequent imaging is directed by clinical suspicion of recurrence.

Tip

- CT has the advantage of detecting calcification within the tumour and this is usually visible on the post-contrast-enhanced CT images, obviating the need for non-contrast CT images (to keep the radiation burden to a minimum).

Rhabdomyosarcoma

Clinical background

Rhabdomyosarcoma is the third commonest soft tissue tumour of childhood following Wilms' tumour and neuroblastoma. Most rhabdomyosarcoma occurs in the head and neck region and in the pelvis. Rhabdomyosarcoma is usually chemo-sensitive, and sometimes there is no residual mass on cross-sectional imaging following treatment.

Who should be imaged?

On discovery of a mass likely to be rhabdomyosarcoma, the primary tumour should be imaged using MRI of the appropriate body part in all patients. There is a high incidence of metastasis at the time of diagnosis and all patients should be subjected to full staging, most easily achieved with CT.

Staging objectives

- To define extent of local disease. Bulky masses may be present and metastasise to regional lymph nodes (cervical for head and neck rhabdomyosarcoma, and pelvic and retroperitoneal for pelvic rhabdomyosarcoma).

- Parameningeal spread through the neural foraminae and skull base should be actively sought in head and neck rhabdomyosarcoma.

- Diagnosis for distant metastatic disease which is seen in up to 10-18% of patients at the time of diagnosis, most frequently to lung, bone and liver.

Staging

MRI

MRI is the preferred technique for imaging head and neck rhabdomyosarcoma owing to its greater sensitivity for detection of parameningeal spread and greater accuracy in discriminating tumour from retained secretions in paranasal sinuses.

Protocol for imaging of neuroblastoma				
Coil	Sequence	Plane	Slice thickness	Field of view
Head or neck	T1W	Coronal	6 ± 2 mm	To fit the body part
Head or neck	T2W	Coronal	6 ± 2 mm	To fit the body part
Head or neck	T1W	Axial	6 ± 2 mm	To fit the body part
Head or neck	T2W	Axial	6 ± 2 mm	To fit the body part
Head or neck	STIR	Coronal – whole neck for detection of nodes		To fit the body part

MRI is also the preferred technique for imaging rhabdomyosarcoma tumours elsewhere, particularly for pelvic, paraspinal and extremity tumours. For pelvic and abdominal rhabdomyosarcoma, MRI or CT may be adequate.

Protocol for imaging of pelvic rhabdomyosarcoma				
Coil	Sequence	Plane	Slice thickness	Field of view
Pelvic / abdominal	T1W	Coronal	6 ± 2 mm	To fit patient
Pelvic / abdominal	T2W	Coronal	6 ± 2 mm	To fit patient
Pelvic / abdominal	T1W	Axial	6 ± 2 mm	To fit patient
Pelvic / abdominal	T2W	Axial	6 ± 2 mm	To fit patient
Pelvic / abdominal	STIR	Coronal – whole pelvis for detection of nodes		To fit patient

For detection of pulmonary, nodal and hepatic disease, a combination of US and CT is adequate. Radionuclide bone scanning is performed routinely in all patients at diagnosis. MRI may be more sensitive in demonstrating bone metastases if there is a clinical history suggestive of bone involvement.

CT

CT scans should be obtained through the region of primary tumour and the chest following the injection of IV contrast medium.

- Dosage of IV contrast medium is 1 ml/0.5 kg patient body weight with scanning at 65-70 seconds post-injection.
- Using MDCT, slice thickness will depend on scanner capability. In general, sections are acquired at 1.25-2.5 mm and reformatted at 5 mm for viewing.

Values of $CTDI_{vol}$ should normally be below the relevant national reference dose for the region of scan and patient group (see Appendix and section on *Radiation Protection for the Patient in CT* in chapter 2).

Follow-up

Repeat imaging after neoadjuvant chemotherapy is used to plan further management. Local recurrence after surgery or radiotherapy is not infrequent, and a post-treatment baseline is useful for further follow-up which is usually precipitated by recurrent local symptoms.

Tip

- In initial investigation of an abdominal soft tissue mass, identification of the organ of origin is a very important first step. Current staging of Wilms' tumour and neuroblastoma take into account surgical / pathological findings.

CHAPTER 22

Malignant melanoma

Clinical background

The incidence of malignant melanoma continues to increase and occurs most frequently in fair-skinned people with a significant history of sun exposure. The majority of patients presenting with a pigmented mole are treated by surgical excision and require no imaging. Some definitions concerning lymph node spread are useful; satellite lesions are defined as lymphatic metastases within 2 cm of the primary lesion, and in-transit metastases occur more than 2 cm from the primary lesion but before the first echelon of the regional lymph nodes. Patients who may require staging investigation by CT include those with in-transit metastases, regional nodal metastases or distant metastases, and those with poor prognosis primary melanomas as defined by primary tumour depth or the presence of lesion ulceration. Malignant melanoma may metastasise widely, including to the liver, lung and brain; there may be multiple soft tissue nodules and bowel metastases, as well. Patients with regional nodal metastases usually undergo radical dissection. Patients may be offered adjuvant biological or chemotherapy. The AJCC staging system for melanoma (2001) is used in the UK guidelines. They emphasise melanoma thickness and ulceration of the primary lesion and the number and clinical presence (occult or macroscopic) of regional lymph nodes.

Who should be imaged?

Those patients with no clinical evidence of regional or distant metastasis with "low risk" for metastasis or melanoma-specific mortality (i.e., Stage I defined histologically – 2 mm or less no ulceration, less than 1 mm with ulceration) require no imaging. Stage II patients are at "intermediate risk" (greater in depth and in degree of ulceration than stage I but with no involvement of regional lymph nodes) and should be considered for a baseline liver ultrasound and CXR. Patients with Stage III/IV disease (distant metastases) are examined with CT of liver, lungs and regional nodal sites and CXR (head and neck, upper limb and torso melanoma patients do not require imaging of the pelvis).

Staging objectives

- To detect macroscopic lymphadenopathy (location, number or in-transit).
- To detect distant visceral metastases.
- To assess other sites of involvement suspected clinically.

Metastases

CT

CT is the preferred technique for staging.

- Chest, abdomen and pelvis (to cover the groin area) for primary staging of lower limb or lower body wall primary tumours.
- Chest and abdomen for upper limb, neck and upper torso primary tumours.
- Oral administration of 1 litre of water or iodinated contrast medium.
- 100-150 ml of intravenous iodinated contrast medium injected at 3-4 ml/sec.
- MDCT is commenced at 20-25 seconds (chest) and 70-80 seconds (abdomen and pelvis) post-injection.
- Using MDCT, slice thickness will depend on scanner capability. In general, sections are acquired at 1.25-2.5 mm and reformatted at 5 mm for viewing.
- Some chemotherapy regimens require exclusion of brain metastases before treatment in view of brain toxicity. Examination of the brain immediately following contrast medium examination with CT suffices.

There is no case for routine examination of the neck as it has not been shown to modify surgical management. However, melanoma may present at a variety of sites within the head and neck including the sinonasal spaces and orbit. Imaging with either CT and / or MRI should be tailored to the treatment plan in each case.

The chest is examined using a protocol for detection of lung metastases and in the arterial phase to maximise detection of mediastinal and hilar nodal metastases. The liver, upper abdomen and pelvis, when indicated, are examined using a portal venous phase protocol for metastases.

Values of $CTDI_{vol}$ should normally be below the relevant national reference dose for the region of scan and patient group (see Appendix and section on *Radiation Protection for the Patient in CT* in chapter 2).

PET-CT

Metastatic malignant melanoma takes up [18]FDG avidly and therefore [18]FDG PET-CT is a powerful technique for detecting and staging metastatic disease. It is particularly useful for detecting occult sites of metastatic disease, for example, intramuscular and bone deposits. [18]FDG PET-CT is not appropriate for the detection of brain metastases due to physiological uptake of [18]FDG by the brain.

119

Follow-up

There is no place for routine follow-up of patients with Stage I / II disease.

For monitoring of treatment response in patients with Stage III and IV disease repeat imaging as in the initial staging scan. The brain examination may be omitted after the initial exclusion of metastasis. Protocols may be modified in clinical trials.

Tips

- A CXR in patients with pulmonary metastases may be useful as a method of follow-up.

- There may be an indeterminate mass in the neck, groin or axilla on CT staging examinations performed soon after nodal dissection. This may comprise haemorrhage, which usually resolves in follow-up, or a myocutaneous graft which may result in a persistent mass. Long-term scarring after surgery is also common. If there is clinical doubt about the presence of active disease within these areas of scarring, then [18]FDG PET-CT scans can be helpful.

- Ultrasound of the inguinal nodes may be helpful in patients with lower limb in-transit metastases.

- MRI may be helpful for characterising melanoma metastases as the paramagnetic effect of melanin results in high signal intensity on T1W images and low / intermediate signal intensity on T2W images. This can be helpful for evaluating patients with indeterminate liver, lung and nodal lesions.

CHAPTER 23

Carcinoma of unknown primary origin

Clinical background

The incidence of carcinoma of unknown primary (CUP) or occult primary origin ranges from 0.5-9% of all patients diagnosed with cancer. Identification of the primary lesion largely forms the basis for predicting the expected behaviour and for assigning appropriate therapy of the malignant disease; thus the identification of a primary tumour poses a major challenge. The most common histology is adenocarcinoma (well- to moderately-differentiated 50%; undifferentiated 30%), squamous cell cancer (15%) and undifferentiated cancer (5%). There is considerable controversy over the extent of evaluation needed to locate a primary cancer. A limited diagnostic approach aiming to recognise patients with good prognostic features is considered the best approach. Histological analysis of biopsy material with immuno-histochemistry establishes the diagnosis and helps to direct further investigations.

Critically, it is important to identify a subset of patients with highly treatable malignancies (e.g., lymphoma, neuroendocrine, breast and primary germ cell tumours). These subsets include:

- Patients present with squamous cancer involving cervical lymph nodes.
- Women with isolated axillary nodal enlargement.
- Women with peritoneal carcinomatosis of papillary adenocarcinoma histology.
- Poorly-differentiated and undifferentiated carcinomas (comprising lymphoma, germ cell neoplasms or neuroendocrine tumours).
- Isolated inguinal nodal enlargement from squamous cell carcinoma.
- Metastatic melanoma to a single nodal site.
- Patients with a single small metastasis.

Who should be imaged?

All patients with suspected or diagnosed carcinoma in whom the origin of the primary tumour is unknown.

Staging objectives

- To identify the full extent of disease and guide the selection of the optimal site for biopsy.

- To identify the site of the primary tumour in order to assign the appropriate therapy.

- To determine potentially favourable subsets of patients with highly treatable malignancies.

The appropriate use of imaging is dependent principally on distribution and histology of known disease. The distribution of disease can provide clues to the likelihood of the primary site being above or below the diaphragm. Lung metastases are twice as common in primary sites ultimately found to be above the diaphragm. Liver metastases are more common from primary disease below the diaphragm. When evaluating patients it is important to remember that the pattern of metastatic spread of a cancer presenting as an occult lesion can be significantly different from that which would be expected from the usual presentation. For example, bone metastases are approximately 3 times more common in pancreatic cancer presenting as occult lesions, but for lung cancer bone metastases are about 10 times less common.

Metastatic squamous cancer of the neck

Most patients presenting with metastatic squamous cancer to the neck will present with cervical lymphadenopathy and 85% will have a squamous cell cancer of the aero-digestive tract. For these patients, either a contrast-enhanced CT or MRI scan and panendoscopy are required to identify the primary tumour. CT should also include the chest as otherwise occult primary lung cancer may also present with metastatic nodal disease in the neck. When a metastatic squamous tumour is found within neck lymph nodes and routine imaging, panendoscopy and biopsy are all negative, an [18]FDG PET-CT scan is indicated for locating the primary tumour. Asymmetric uptake of [18]FDG on PET-CT of the tonsils should be considered with suspicion.

Values of $CTDI_{vol}$ should normally be below the relevant national reference dose for the region of scan and patient group (see Appendix and section on *Radiation Protection for the Patient in CT* in chapter 2).

Metastatic adenocarcinoma of unknown primary origin

CT scans of the abdomen and pelvis together with a CXR or CT are indicated in most patients but will result in the detection of a primary site in 30-35% of patients. It should be noted that in 15-25% of patients, the primary site cannot be identified even at post-mortem examination. The diagnostic value of [18]FDG PET-CT is not recommended due to the small evidence base.

CT

- Oral administration of 1 litre of water or iodinated contrast medium.

- 100-150 ml IV iodinated contrast medium injected at 3-4 ml/sec.

- MDCT is commenced at 20-25 seconds (chest) and 70-80 seconds (abdomen and pelvis) following injection.

- Using MDCT, slice thickness will depend on scanner capability. In general, sections are acquired at 1.25-2.5 mm and reformatted at 5 mm for viewing.

Values of CTDI$_{vol}$ should normally be below the relevant national reference dose for the region of scan and patient group (see Appendix and section on *Radiation Protection for the Patient in CT* in chapter 2).

Follow-up

Is conducted to assess response to chemotherapy and is therefore performed at a frequency to correspond with the chemotherapy regimens.

Metastatic neuroendocrine tumour

There are three clinico-pathological subtypes described: low-grade tumours such as well-differentiated carcinoid or Islet cell tumours which usually involve the liver; small cell anaplastic carcinoma; and poorly differentiated tumours with immunohistochemical staining suggestive of neuroendocrine origin. CT scans of the abdomen and pelvis together with a CXR or CT are indicated in most patients, but the primary tumour is often not found.

Tip

- For the special cases of metastatic adenocarcinoma within axillary lymph nodes with negative clinical and mammographic findings (whatever the hormonal status), an MRI examination of both breasts with contrast enhancement is indicated.

123

CHAPTER 24

Breast cancer

Clinical background

At the time of diagnosis of breast cancer, the investigations commonly used, i.e., mammography and ultrasound, together with clinical examination and histology will establish local disease stage. The size of the primary tumour will guide choice of therapy; early breast cancer may be treated with surgery while more locally advanced tumours will often be treated with neoadjuvant chemotherapy prior to surgery in an attempt to downsize local disease and reduce the requirement for mastectomy.

Patients with T1 and T2 primary breast tumours (i.e., less than 5 cm) have a low incidence of distant metastatic disease at the time of diagnosis of less than 2%. Patients presenting with T3 and T4 tumours have an incidence of metastatic disease at the time of diagnosis of between 15-20%. Overall, approximately 4% of patients presenting with breast cancer will have metastatic disease detectable at the time of diagnosis. In patients with T1 and T2 tumours, screening for asymptomatic metastases is difficult to justify on clinical grounds and generates false positive findings. Detection of metastases at an asymptomatic stage in bone and CNS has not been shown to prolong survival.

Who should be imaged?

"Routine" CT staging for asymptomatic patients with early stage disease (T1 / T2) is not indicated. If symptoms develop, the appropriate investigation should be requested. Even in patients with advanced disease (T3 / T4), including inflammatory carcinoma, routine CT is not generally done. A bone scan with liver ultrasound is performed first by most centres. Breast MRI scanning should be considered in patients suspected to have multifocal / multicentric cancer where the treatment strategy may be altered (e.g., when breast conservation would be preferred) particularly for large tumours in the radiographically dense breast and for lobular cancers. MRI should also be considered to identify the extent of residual cancer if positive surgical margins are found following

Staging objectives

- To establish size of tumour.

- To assess for skin and chest wall involvement.

- To assess for multifocality and multicentricity of tumour.

- To establish nodal status with respect to nodal involvement and anatomical site.

- To assess for distant metastatic disease in patients who are symptomatic or considered at unusually high risk of having metastatic disease.

Staging

Diagnostic investigations for breast cancer include ultrasound and mammography. Fine needle aspiration for cytological examination or core biopsy is almost always used to confirm the suspected clinical diagnosis. These diagnostic investigations may then be used for staging local disease. Mammography is able to detect calcification with greater sensitivity than ultrasound, while axillary nodal status is assessed better with ultrasound. There is frequently some discrepancy between the estimated tumour dimensions on clinical examination, ultrasound and mammography, and all 3 techniques should be taken into consideration before assigning local disease stage.

MRI

MRI is the most sensitive method of detecting multifocal invasive carcinoma and is used in selected cases. Clinical indications for staging breast MRI include suspected multiple bilateral tumours and positive surgical margins following breast conservation surgery. CT does not have a role in staging primary disease, and the use of [18]FDG PET-CT is experimental. Sentinel node imaging at the time of surgery is now widely used. However, the methods used vary widely and not all surgeons consider the technique useful.

Single dose contrast 0.2ml/kg patient body weight. Temporal resolution of each dynamic scan not more than 90 seconds.

Protocol for breast imaging

Sequence	Plane	Slice thickness	Field of view
TSE T2W	Transverse	4 mm x 0	Both breasts
TSE T2W	Sagittal	4 mm x 0	Affected breast
Dynamic contrast-enhanced T1 gradient echo + Fat Sat x 6	Sagittal	4 mm x 0	Affected breast
Delayed T1 gradient echo + Fat Sat Post-contrast	Sagittal	4 mm x 0	Affected breast

125

CT

"Routine" staging for asymptomatic patients with early stage disease is not indicated. If symptoms develop, the appropriate investigation should be requested (e.g., for bone pain, isotope bone imaging; for breathlessness, CXR initially and thoracic CT, if radiograph is normal and lymphangitis is suspected; and for symptomatic brachial plexopathy, MRI is the preferred investigation). If staging CT scanning is performed, the supraclavicular fossa, chest and liver should be examined using IV contrast medium.

- 100-150 ml of IV iodinated contrast medium injected at 3-4 ml/sec.
- MDCT is commenced at 20-25 seconds (neck and chest) and 70-80 seconds (abdomen and pelvis) following injection.
- Using MDCT, slice thickness will depend on scanner capability. In general, sections are acquired at 1.25-2.5 mm and reformatted at 5 mm for viewing.

Values of $CTDI_{vol}$ should normally be below the relevant national reference dose for the region of scan and patient group (see Appendix and section on *Radiation Protection for the Patient in CT* in chapter 2).

PET-CT

[18]FDG PET-CT is not routinely indicated for primary tumour / axillary staging because its accuracy is limited. [18]FDG PET-CT is becoming recognised as the most accurate imaging modality for detecting metastatic disease recurrence and it is particularly useful for the definition of small volume (less than 1 cm) involved nodal disease and lytic bone metastases. The modality is currently used predominantly for the assessment of patients with equivocal imaging or clinical findings, frequently providing a definitive assessment regarding the presence or absence of active recurrent metastatic disease.

Follow-up

Imaging of the treated breast following surgery may be undertaken with mammography or ultrasound. Although interpretation may be hampered by post-operative scarring and radiation change, mammography can be expected to detect 30-40% of clinically occult recurrence. Mammography is also useful for confirming the absence of recurrence. Ultrasound may be used to attempt to characterise areas of breast with palpable abnormality following treatment and to guide fine needle aspiration for cytology or repeat biopsy. There is no clear evidence on the optimum interval for performing follow-up mammography or ultrasound.

Following diagnosis of breast cancer, the patient is at increased risk of developing carcinoma in the contralateral breast. 80% of contralateral breast cancers will have arisen within 10 years of treatment of the first cancer; the remaining 20% of contralateral cancers arise over the following 15 years. The surveillance interval should take this into account.

Tips

- There is no demonstrable survival benefit derived from intensive imaging follow-up aimed at early detection of metastases in asymptomatic patients.
- Follow-up imaging after treatment for non-metastatic breast cancer should be directed by clinical symptoms.

Appendix:

National reference values of CTDI$_{vol}$

National reference doses represent a practical tool for facilitating the optimisation of patient protection.[1] They are specified for CT in terms of two special dose quantities: volume weighted CT dose index (CTDI$_{vol}$), which represents the average dose to the scanned volume of a standard CT dosimetry phantom for a particular scan sequence; and dose-length product (DLP), which takes account of the volume of irradiation so as to represent the total energy imparted by the examination. National reference values for these doses are based on the third quartiles of the distributions observed in periodic national reviews of practice and, as such, provide a simple yardstick for identifying centres where levels of dose are unusually high. Any technique for which doses are above the relevant national reference dose should be critically reviewed and either clinically justified or revised so as to reduce patient doses without loss of clinical efficacy.

National reference doses for CTDI$_{vol}$ published following the 2003 UK review of CT are summarised in Tables 1 and 2 for examinations on adult and paediatric patients respectively.[1] Separate values are shown for examinations on adults with multi-slice (MDCT) and single-slice (SSCT) CT scanners, although general values are given for paediatric CT; the doses for examinations of the adult head and children relate to the 16 cm diameter CT dosimetry phantom, whereas those of the adult trunk relate to the 32 cm diameter CT dosimetry phantom. Such national reference doses will be updated periodically on the basis of further timely national reviews of CT practice. Whereas the national reference values for CTDI$_{vol}$ in Tables 1 and 2 can be applied to the imaging tasks in this document, there is presently a lack of appropriate values of DLP for the general scanning techniques described.

Values of CTDI$_{vol}$ should be assessed for each CT protocol, from the scanner display, where available and validated, or by calculation.[1] In the first instance, local levels should normally be below any national reference dose relevant to the scan region. However, since such reference values are clearly not optimum doses, further dose reductions should always be pursued, where clinically compatible, in close collaboration with medical physics experts.

Table 1: UK national reference doses (2003) for single slice (SSCT) and multislice (MSCT) CT on adult patients.[1]

Scan region	2003 National reference value for CTDI$_{vol}$ (mGy)	
	SSCT	MSCT
Head (posterior fossa)	65	100
Head (cerebrum)	55	65
Thorax	10	13
Abdomen or pelvis	13	14

Table 2: General UK national reference doses (2003) for CT on paediatric patients.[1]

Patient group	Scan region	2003 National reference value for CTDI$_{vol}$ (mGy)
0-1 year old	Head (posterior fossa)	35
	Head (cerebrum)	**30**
	Thorax	12
5 year old	Head (posterior fossa)	50
	Head (cerebrum)	45
	Thorax	13
10 year old	Head (posterior fossa)	65
	Head (cerebrum)	50
	Thorax	20

Reference

1. Shrimpton P C, Hillier M C, Lewis M A and Dunn M (2005). Doses from computed tomography (CT) examinations in the UK – 2003 review. Chilton, NRPB-W67. Available online via Health Protection Agency website:

http://www.hpa.org.uk/radiation/publications/w_series_reports/2005/nrpb_w67.htm.